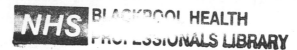

Surgical MCQs

For Churchill Livingstone

Publisher: Laurence Hunter
Project Editor: Dilys Jones
Production Controller: Lesley W. Small, Debra L. Barrie
Sales Promotion Executive: Marion Pollock

Surgical MCQs

J. L. Craven
BSc MD FRCS
Consultant Surgeon, York District Hospital

J. S. P. Lumley
MS FRCS
Professor of Vascular Surgery and Honorary
Consultant in Surgery, St Bartholomew's Hospital,
London

THIRD EDITION

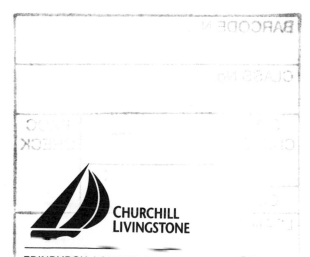

CHURCHILL
LIVINGSTONE

EDINBURGH LONDON NEW YORK PHILADELPHIA SYDNLY
TORONTO 1993

CHURCHILL LIVINGSTONE
An imprint of Harcourt Publishers Limited

© Longman Group Limited 1976, 1985
© Longman Group UK Limited 1993
© Harcourt Brace and Company Limited 1999
© Harcourt Publishers Limited 2001

 is a registered trademark of Harcourt Publishers Limited

First edition 1976
Second edition 1985
Third edition 1993
  Reprinted 1996
  Reprinted 1998
  Reprinted 1999
  Reprinted 2001

ISBN 0 443 04702 2

British Library Cataloguing in Publication Data
A catalogue record for this book is available from the
British Library

Library of Congress Cataloging in Publication Data
A catalog record for this book is available
from the Library of Congress

Printed in China by RDC Group Limited
B/05

Contents

Preface

An examination system which is to assess the results of a number of years of study should do so fairly, uniformly and reliably; it should cover as much of the syllabus as possible, and be able to differentiate between good and bad candidates in a consistent manner. The objective test succeeds to a large degree in fulfilling these requirements but in itself it must not be a handicap to the candidate who should be well versed in this form of examination technique.

It is not claimed that the questions in the subsequent chapters will provide a painless method of passing the undergraduate's surgical finals, for it is hoped that the horizon of examining boards will include data obtained from other important spheres such as continuous assessment, long term case studies, oral assessment and conventional essay-style questions. It is hoped that the book will provide the student with an introduction to objective testing and, in particular, with a method of both testing and improving his surgical knowledge.

This new edition has provided an opportunity to update the text, introduce new questions and delete questions which have been found to have poor discriminant powers.

A fifth option has also been added to each question, in keeping with the format of most undergraduate and postgraduate medical examinations.

A series of self-assessment questions has been included at the end of the text. In this chapter no explanations are given for the answers. However, as these questions are based on earlier material, if problems arise, the reader can refer back to the appropriate chapter for further clarification.

1993   J.L.C.
                                                                        J.S.P.L.

Introduction

Objective Testing

The perfect examination would be one in which the student was accurately assessed in his knowledge, comprehension, application, analysis and evaluation of material pertinent to the subject being examined. The use of the essay type question paper as the sole means of assessment has been criticised because of its reliance on subjective (and therefore unmeasurable) qualities.

For several years educationalists of many different disciplines have sought methods of objective testing which examined all the above mentioned qualities. In all objective tests the student has to choose the correct response out of one or more alternatives, his answers being either right or wrong. The subjective judgement of the examiner thus plays no part in this form of examination. Objective testing has been used extensively in the USA since the end of the Second World War, but Introduction in the UK was slow, and it reached the universities generally via schools and technical colleges. However, a multiple choice question paper is now in use in most undergraduate and postgraduate medical examinations and it is necessary for both the student and the medical teacher to become fully acquainted with the uses and abuses of this testing technique. It is appropriate here to consider the merits of the various examination techniques and, perhaps most important, to compare objective testing with the traditional essay question.

The Essay

Students and examiners have questioned the effectiveness of an essay paper in measuring the attainment of a number of years of study. The area covered by such an examination is very limited, the more so when a wide choice of questions is allowed. It thus encourages the students to 'spot questions' and to concentrate on only part of the syllabus. The marking of essays is time consuming and unreliable, there being marked variations in an individual examiner's reassessment of papers as well as between examiners. This variation makes comparison on a national level difficult and is further accentuated by what has been described as the deep psychological barrier of examiners to allocate more than seventy per cent of the total marks allowed for any given essay question. However, the essay does determine the candidate's ability to write clear and legible English, it tests his ability to collect and quantitate material and it assesses his powers of logic, original thought and creativity. In terms of cost the essay question is cheap to produce but it is expensive to mark.

The Composition of Objective Questions

The objective form of examination is best composed by a panel of examiners, each having a complete understanding of the syllabus and a thorough knowledge of the field of study. The panel must first decide the parts of the syllabus to be covered by the examination, and the level of knowledge required by the candidate. The type of objective test and the number of options per question is decided and each member of the panel prepares a set of questions for the group to consider. A multiple choice question consists of a stem (the initial question) and four or more options; one of these options in the multiple choice question is correct and this is known as the key, the incorrect responses being known as the distractors. In the case of multiple response questions, there may be more than one correct response. (This form of question has also been termed multiple completion, multiple answer, multiple true or false and the indeterminate response by various authorities, but in most centres, and in this test, it will subsequently be referred to as a multiple choice question.)

Stem and options should be brief using the minimum number of words and the instructions should be clear and simple, the language used being appropriate to the verbal ability and requirement of the candidate. The questions must always be some educational value. The words 'always' and 'never' should be avoided and the stem should preferably not be in the negative. There should be no recurrent phrase in the options which can be included in the stem. The key (the correct option or options) must be wholly correct and unambiguous. It is important for the correct response to be in different positions in each of a group of questions and some form of random allocation may be necessary. The distractors (the wrong options) are the most exacting and challenging part of objective question composition and the standard of an objective test is probably best assessed in terms of the quality of its distractors. They must always be plausible, yet completely wrong. They should be in a parallel style to the key and they should not contain clues. Common misconceptions form good distractors. 'None of them' or 'all of them' are not satisfactory distractors.

After the draft questions have been collected, it is advisable for a panel of examiners to assess their value and limitations. Inaccurate and irrelevant material is then excluded. Even the most experienced of examiners will find that a panel will offer constructive criticism on the majority of his questions. Ideally, once the panel has accepted a series of questions these should be pre-tested on a group of students and the results analysed. It is desirable for a question to have been pre-tested on 300 to 400 students before it comes into regular use in a qualifying examination. The difficulty of a question can be determined by calculating the percentage of students giving the right answer, and its discriminatory value (the ratio of correct/incorrect responses) calculated in a manner which takes into account whether or not the better students obtained the correct response. The facility value (difficulty index) records the percentage of correct responses and compares it with the total number of candidates. Additional information on the mean range of distribution of the answers can also be obtained with a discriminatory index and a bi-serial correlation coefficient (relating the total candidate response to an option, with the results of the top 27 per cent and the bottom 27 per cent of the candidates to the same option). Figures for both the discriminatory index and the bi-serial correlation coefficient range from plus 1 to minus 1. Questions with factors of less than 0.20 should be rejected (unless a few difficult or easy questions are to be included). Values of 0.21 to 0.39 show a reasonable discriminatory power of the option, whereas results greater than 0.44 indicate good discrimination by a question of the candidates under test. The effectiveness of the question is also measured in terms of the number of students attempting it – the value of a question certainly cannot be assessed if a large number of students leave it out. Computer readouts on a series of questions will also provide the ranking of students, the scatter of the results and a raw score (i.e. the number of correct less the number of incorrect results).

The pre-testing, though very time consuming, greatly adds to the validity and reliability of the objective test. Using the results of these tests the panel can rephrase unsatisfactory questions and compile the definitive examination paper. The time allowed in the pre-test is not limited but the students are asked to note the time taken to complete the test; the time required for the final version is thus arrived at. This time should allow at least 90 per cent of the candidates to complete the paper. It is usual to start an examination paper with a few easier questions (i.e. with a low difficulty index) and similarly a few difficult questions can be included at the end. It has been found that a good (wide) range of results is obtained by setting a large number of questions with average discrimination rather than including a large number with high or low discriminatory indices. Testing of the questions should not stop after the pre-testing phase, the information gained from each subsequent examination should be used to continuously review all the question material.

Obviously a series of questions which have been pre-tested and shown to be satisfactory is of great value to the examiner. Such questions can be used repeatedly provided they have not been freely available to the student. Security is an important factor, particularly when the number of questions is small and does not cover the whole syllabus. For this reason it is advisable to have a large number of questions available. It is reasonable to assume that if a student is capable of memorising the correct responses to a large number of questions (even if these are known to him) he will also have a passable knowledge of the syllabus.

A satisfactory bank of questions takes 3 to 5 years to build. After this time the questions can be grouped into sections and, whenever an examination paper is required, questions can be chosen at random from each section. Continuous updating and revision of this material should be undertaken and new material added regularly. The history of each question in the bank should be recorded. Repetitive use of the questions over a number of years allows annual standards to be compared.

The Student's Approach To Objective Testing

Any student required to undertake an objective test for a qualifying examination or postgraduate examination should ensure he has some preliminary experience in this form of testing. It is essential for him to know and have sampled the style of questions used by his particular examining board.

In any objective test all the instructions provided must be carefully read and understood and the student's designated number marked in the appropriate section, otherwise a computer marking system will reject the paper – this will not impress the examining authority.

The type of objective test used in medical education does vary and some of these types have already been discussed. Whatever form the question takes in the objective test it is essential that the student starts on his first quick 'run' through the questions by filling in all the answers he knows to be correct. On this first 'run' he should also mark (on the paper) the questions where he is fully acquainted with the material but is unsure of the correct response. On the second 'run' all his attention can now be given to the latter group of questions, in which he should be able to make an informed guess. Experience has shown that his chances of being correct in this situation are above average. He should, as one examiner expresses it, 'play his hunches'. The questions which he does not understand are probably best left unanswered as at best he can only hope for a 50 per cent chance of a correct response on a random basis in the true/false situation, and only a 25 per cent chance of a correct response in a four-item multiple choice question. In multiple choice questions the marking is usually positive, a mark being given for a correct answer and none for an incorrect one. In multiple response questions (as in this text) a mark is given for each correct response, whether this be true or false, and usually a mark is subtracted for each incorrect response. Most examination systems have now abolished the use of a correction factor for guessing as this was found to have little effect on the ranking of the candidates; it has also been realised that informed guessing is in itself a useful discrimination.

Lack of time is not usually a problem in medical objective testing. These tests are of the 'power' rather than the 'speed' variety, i.e. knowledge rather than ability against the clock is being tested. Excessive time may be a disadvantage to the candidate as repeated reassessment of the answers may distract from the correct response rather than produce improvement. In the multiple choice situation it has been found that 1 minute is usually necessary per question although more time is required to answer a question containing a number of distractors.

Transcribing 300 items from a question paper to an answer sheet (i.e. 60 questions each with 5 options) takes a minimum of 10 minutes and the habit of leaving such transcriptions to the end of an examination is best avoided since, if rushed, it may introduce unnecessary inaccuracies.

Etymological Hazards

The rarity of absolutes in medicine means that a large variety of adjectives and adverbs are commonly used in its description. These increase the difficulty of both setting and answering multiple choice questions. Although one can question the desirability of assessing knowledge which is dependent on the 'strength of an adjective', these adjectives do form the language of present day medical practice. This factor is borne out by their frequent use in the questions and answers of the present text. Nevertheless, the examiner must avoid ambiguity and in addition his questions must not contain clues to the correct answer. Such terms as 'invariable', 'always', 'must', 'all', 'only', and 'never' should be avoided since they imply absolutes and are therefore likely to be wrong.

The terms 'may' and 'can' also give rise to ambiguity. In medicine almost anything 'may occur' and statements using this phrase are unlikely to be completely wrong. If these terms are used and the student is able to answer that the question 'certainly may' or 'certainly may not', he has little chance of being wrong. The term 'sometimes' comes into the same category.

The adjectives and adverbs 'common', 'usual', 'frequent' (commonly, usually, frequently), 'likely' and 'often' are an integral part of everyday medical language but their use in the multiple choice question may also lead to ambiguity. Their meanings are very similar yet their values depend largely on the context of the question. Expressed as incidences they may well range from 30 to 70 per cent. They may be considerably modified by the addition of 'quite', 'most', 'very' and 'extremely'. The examiner must be particularly careful of his choice of these terms. The 'majority' implies more than 50 per cent, whereas the 'vast majority' implies nearly 100 per cent.

The term 'typical' is a useful one for multiple choice questions. Its meaning implies 'that which is found in clinical practice'. 'Characteristic' implies a time honoured diagnostic feature and 'recognised' an accepted text book feature. Less explicit, and therefore less desirable, terminology includes 'most authorities agree', 'generally assumed', 'probable', 'thought to be', 'all reports indicate' and 'has recently been reported'. Further vague terminology used in medical practice yet best avoided in the multiple choice situation includes 'associated with', 'accompanied by', 'related to', 'linked with' and 'lend support to'.

On the negative side, 'uncommon', 'unusual', 'infrequent' (uncommonly, unusually, infrequently), 'unlikely' and 'rare' are all terms commonly used yet their use in the multiple choice situation must not give rise to ambiguity. As with their positive equivalents they are markedly influenced by the addition of such terms as 'most' and 'very'. The term 'significant' is best kept for its statistical use and the terms 'increased' and 'more' should be restricted to direct comparative situations.

The terms 'demand' and 'should' indicate the examiner's personal opinion and, although their inclusion is questionable, the student is still required to indicate whether he thinks the opinion is valid.

In conclusion, words used in multiple choice questions, although giving rise to apparent ambiguity, remain those in common use in medical practice; both the examiner and the student must be fully conversant with their meanings and disadvantages in order to avoid any confusion. It is hoped that the questions which follow will also help in this regard.

How to use this book

The text, consisting of questions and answers ('true or false'), is arranged throughout in such a way that all questions appear on left-hand pages and all answers on right-hand pages.

In use the student may conveniently cover the right-hand page with a blank sheet on which to jot down his answers for comparison.

1 Fluid and electrolyte balance

1 **The normal adult value for**
   A urine output is 1.5 litre/day
   B insensible water loss is 200 ml/day
   C potassium requirement is 150 mEq (150 mmol)/day
   D protein requirement is 70 g/day
   E serum albumin is 35 g/litre

2 **In a healthy 70 kg male the**
   A total body water measures approximately 40 litres
   B extracellular fluid volume measures approximately 8 litres
   C plasma volume measures approximately 3.5 litres
   D 'third space' fluid measures approximately 1 litre
   E resting energy expenditure decreases postoperatively

1   A   **True**   In a temperate climate.
    B   **False**   Insensible loss via skin and lungs ranges from 700 to
                    1000 ml/day and will be increased during fever and
                    high ambient temperatures.
    C   **False**   Potassium requirements of the healthy adult are 40
                    to 60 mEq (40 to 60 mmol)/day. There are excessive
                    losses during starvation, hypercatabolic states,
                    intestinal obstruction and diarrhoea.
    D   **True**   This is increased in hypercatabolic states such as
                    burns and severe sepsis.
    E   **True**   Decreased in starvation.

2   A   **True**   The average values are 62 per cent of total body
                    weight in males and 52 per cent in females.
    B   **False**   The extracellular fluid volume measures about 22 per
                    cent of the body weight, i.e. approximately 15 litres.
                    This includes plasma volume, lymph and interstitial
                    fluid.
    C   **True**   The whole blood volume being approximately 5
                    litres.
    D   **True**   This is the fluid normally in the pleural and peritoneal
                    cavities and the cerebrospinal fluid together with the
                    secretions in the alimentary tract. This component
                    enlarges considerably at the expense of the
                    extracellular fluid volume in peritonitis, intestinal
                    obstruction and with any large inflammatory area.
    E   **False**   Trauma, sickness and postoperative convalescence
                    all increase resting energy expenditure from 10 to 40
                    per cent.

3 **The pH of the extracellular fluid**
   A   is maintained in health between 7.4 and 7.6
   B   is maintained entirely by the buffering system of the intra-
       and extracellular fluids
   C   is increased in hypovolaemic shock
   D   decreases abruptly after a cardiac arrest
   E   should be monitored in a critically ill patient

4 **A low serum sodium level**
   A   is commonly present in the early postoperative period
   B   may cause stupor and fits
   C   should be treated with isotonic saline infusions
   D   is associated with an impaired ability to excrete water
   E   is associated with diuretic therapy

5 **The sodium ion is**
   A   the principal regulator of the intracellular volume
   B   the major ionic component of the extracellular fluid volume
   C   present in greater concentration in intracellular fluid than
       extracellular fluid
   D   excreted in larger amounts than normal in the early
       postoperative period
   E   lost in great quantities by the patient with pyloric stenosis

3 A **False** In the healthy individual the pH is maintained
  B **False** between 7.35 and 7.42 by the buffering capacity of
the bicarbonate/carbonic acid system, the phosphate
buffer system and the buffering properties of the
serum proteins and haemoglobin. Additional
regulation is by the lungs and kidneys.
  C **False** Shock is always associated with a metabolic acidosis.
  D **True** The absence of tissue perfusion results in a rapid fall
in the pH of the extracellular fluid.
  E **True** Below pH 7.2 there is an increased tendency to
cardiac irregularities.

4 A **True** Increased antidiuretic hormone production occurs
resulting in increased water retention.
  B **True** This complication may be confused with a
cerebrovascular accident.
  C **False** 3 per cent (hypertonic) saline should be administered
  D **True** in order to produce a diuresis and overcome the
inability of the kidney to excrete water in
hyponatraemia.
  E **True** All diuretics result in excessive sodium loss which in
the ill patient may result in a low serum sodium.

5 A **True** Because of the low intracellular concentration of
  B **True** sodium, ionic movement of the ion into or out of the
extracellular fluid is accompanied by an immediate
movement of fluid into or out of the intracellular
space.
  C **False** Sodium is almost exclusively an extracellular ion.
  D **False** There is an initial postoperative retention of sodium.
  E **True** Loss of sodium-rich gastric contents results in a
hyponatraemic state in these patients.

6 **Potassium deficiency should be suspected**
   A in cases of paralytic ileus
   B when the patient's reflexes are exaggerated
   C if there is an increase in height and peaking of the T waves of an ECG
   D in alkalotic states
   E in renal failure

7 **Potassium deficiency**
   A can be effectively monitored by the serum potassium levels
   B may render digitalis therapy more dangerous
   C should be treated with an infusion of normal saline with potassium supplements
   D is not usually present in intestinal obstruction
   E is usually present in severely burned patients

8 **The effects of a major extracellular fluid deficiency**
   A include a decreased skin turgor
   B include hypotension
   C include excessive salivation
   D may be corrected by an infusion of isotonic saline
   E may result in decreasing consciousness

6 A **True** Potassium deficiency may be both a cause and an effect of paralytic ileus. A diminished intracellular potassium results in atony of both visceral and skeletal muscles.

B **False** The reflexes are decreased.

C **False** The myocardium is also subject to muscle atony and an ECG shows a prolongation of the Q-T interval, depression of the ST segment and eventual inversion of the T wave.

D **True** When there is excessive chloride loss, potassium excretion rises as the kidney attempts to conserve hydrogen ions.

E **False** Renal failure usually results in an increased serum potassium concentration.

7 A **False** The major store of potassium is intracellular and the serum levels may be normal in the presence of a large intracellular deficit.

B **True** Potassium deficiency enhances the effect of digitalis and dysrhythmias are prone to occur.

C **True** The infusion should not contain more than 40 mEq (40 mmol) of potassium/litre and should usually not be administered at more than 15 mEq (15 mmol) potassium/hour.

D **False** A deficient intake and excessive losses of potassium into the bowel lumen often lead to potassium deficiency in this condition.

E **False** Prerenal failure which commonly accompanies this condition will result in a high serum potassium.

8 A **True** Due to the resultant hypovolaemia.

B **True**

C **False** The mucous membranes are drier than normal.

D **True** This solution and other isotonic electrolyte-containing fluids such as Ringer's lactate are the most effective agents for restoring extracellular fluid.

E **True** Cerebral blood flow is diminished and a semi-comatose state frequently results.

9 **Extracellular fluid losses are often extensive in**
   A intestinal obstruction
   B peritonitis
   C pancreatitis
   D hepatic coma
   E myocardial infarction

10 **Excessive vomiting or loss of gastric secretion by nasogastric suction**
   A produces a metabolic alkalosis
   B results in a low serum potassium
   C may produce renal failure
   D should be treated with isotonic saline infusions
   E may result in hypoproteinaemia

11 **Increases in the extracellular fluid volume can be accurately assessed and fluid overloading avoided by**
   A serum electrolyte determinations
   B the measurement of the central venous pressure (CVP)
   C the measurement of hourly urine volumes
   D serial body weighing
   E serial haemoglobin estimation

9 A **True**   In all these conditions there may be extensive
   B **True**   internal translocations of fluid from the extracellular
   C **True**   compartment to the 'third space' (see Q.2).
   D **False**   In liver failure the extracellular fluid volume is usually
                   increased.
   E **False**   This often results in cardiogenic shock. Though
                   hypotension follows, there is no excess loss of
                   extracellular fluid.

10 A **True**   There is an excessive loss of hydrogen and chloride
   B **True**   ions producing an alkalosis. As the loss of chloride
   C **True**   continues the kidney is unable to reabsorb the
                   tubular sodium and substitutes potassium in the
                   tubular urine. Thus potassium excretion rises and
                   serum potassium falls. The associated loss of fluid
   D **True**   often gives rise to uraemia. These metabolic upsets
                   usually respond to infusions of isotonic saline but
                   occasionally potassium needs to be added.
   E **False**   There is no excessive loss of proteins. The resulting
                   haemoconcentration may cause the serum protein
                   levels to be high.

11 A **False**   Normal values are often found in patients with
                   severe abnormalities of extracellular fluid volume.
   B **False**   In chronic hypervolaemia the CVP may not be raised
                   as the bulk of the fluid will lie in the interstitial space
                   rather than in the plasma.
   C **False**   There is often some associated renal failure.
   D **True**   This investigation will reveal extracellular fluid
                   increases prior to the development of pulmonary and
                   sacral oedema. It is particularly useful in the
                   management of chronic hepatic, renal and cardiac
                   problems. In the acutely fluid depleted patient,
                   however, all these factors (A to D) are helpful in
                   assessing fluid requirements.
   E **False**   This rarely gives an accurate estimation of
                   extracellular fluid volume.

12   Anuria in the postoperative period
A   is defined as the production of less than 500 ml of urine/day
B   should be treated with an initial 'waterload', i.e. a 4 litre fluid infusion
C   is associated with hypernatraemia and dehydration
D   is usually treated by renal dialysis
E   should be managed with, amongst other things, a CVP line

13   The anuric patient
A   should have a fluid intake of 1 to 1.5 litres per day
B   should have no potassium administered
C   is at risk from metabolic alkalosis
D   should be on continuous urinary catheter drainage
E   should not be catheterised

14   Acute post-traumatic renal failure
A   is usually the result of direct crush injuries to the kidneys
B   may be due to hypovolaemia and poor tissue perfusion
C   is particularly associated with crush injuries
D   may be due to kidney damage following tubular obstruction
E   should initially be treated by fluid restriction

12 A **False** This is the definition of oliguria. Anura is defined as the production of less than 100 ml/day.

B **False** In the absence of hypovolaemia immediate fluid restriction should be instituted.

C **False** There is almost always overhydration, relative haemodilution and a low serum sodium level.

D **False** Most patients should have precise fluid therapy based on a policy of replacing only insensible and urinary losses. Cases of refractory renal tubular necrosis may be considered for short term dialysis.

E **True** Hourly urine flows are an important measure of urinary function. A CVP line is essential if fluid replacement is to be given safely in these patients.

---

13 A **False** Only insensible losses should be replaced. These will range from 400 to 700 ml/day.

B **True** A rising serum potassium is one of the more serious effects of anuria. When it rises above 6 mEq (6 mmol)/litre exchange resins should be administered orally or rectally and dialysis considered.

C **False** Metabolic acidosis is almost always present and is due to the accumulation of sulphates and phosphates.

D **False** Catheterisation should be avoided unless specific surgical indications are present.

E **True** Catheterisation is frequently followed by urethritis which may extend to cystitis and other urinary tract infections.

---

14 A **False** Post-traumatic renal failure is the result of poor renal infusion and not of direct renal injuries.

B **True** Any prolonged decrease in extracellular fluid volume

C **True** and tissue perfusion will result in renal dysfunction.

D **True** This may also be due to tubular obstruction by blood pigments following crush injuries, mismatched transfusions or burns.

E **False** It is desirable to give a provocative test, such as 1 litre of dextrose intravenously in 90 minutes where hypovolaemia is suspected. Similarly, the initial treatment of tubular necrosis should include a fluid load and diuretics. Only when these methods fail should fluids be restricted.

15   Intravenous parenteral feeding

A   should deliver at least 2500 calories (10 500J)/day to an adult
B   should deliver at least 10 g of nitrogen (i.e. 66 g of protein)/
day to an adult
C   can be effectively achieved with isotonic solutions
D   is without complications with present day solutions and
methods of administration
E   provides better nutritional support than enteral
supplementation

16   Enteral feeding

A   results in constipation
B   often results in uraemia and dehydration
C   carries the risk of gastric reflux and pulmonary complications
D   is ineffective as a long term method of nutrition
E   should be thought of as 'second best' to intravenous
nutrition

15 A **True**   The ideal solution has not yet been found but the
    B **True**   proteins should be in the form of amino acids and
                   the calorie source as carbohydrate and, to a lesser
                   extent, alcohol. Emulsified fat may also be used.
    C **False**   The tolerable limit for water intake in a sick patient is
                   of the order of 3 litres; thus the solutions used, in
                   order to supply the requisite amount of calories and
                   amino acids, must be hypertonic.
    D **False**   Thrombophlebitis and septicaemia are frequent
                   complications, diminished to some extent by the use
                   of large veins and the use of a scrupulous sterile
                   technique when setting up the infusion.
                   Hyperosmolar coma is occasionally seen.
    E **False**   Enteral feeding, when possible, always achieves
                   better results in nutritional terms than intravenous
                   feeding.

16 A **False**   Diarrhoea is common with hyperosmolar diets. It
                   should be treated by reducing the rate of
                   administration.
    B **True**   The feeds are often hyperosmolar and excessive fluid
                   losses in the faeces and urine may produce prerenal
                   uraemia and dehydration.
    C **True**   Rapid administration of fluid may be accompanied by
                   regurgitation and aspiration of gastric contents.
    D **False**   With due precautions to avoid the above
                   complications, this is a satisfactory method for long
                   term nutrition.
    E **False**   Enteral feeding is much superior to intravenous
                   feeding in terms of nutrition. This, if possible, is the
                   favoured nutritional route.

2 Shock and blood transfusion

17 **'Shock' can be most comprehensively defined as**

A a sudden large volume blood loss
B a diminished effective circulating fluid volume
C a hypotensive state with peripheral vasoconstriction
D an unexpected psychological insult
E inadequate cardiac output

18 **In all forms of shock there is**

A an impairment of cellular oxygenation
B a decreased cardiac output
C a diminished effective circulating fluid volume
D a low central venous pressure (CVP)
E tissue acidosis

19 **The pulmonary insufficiency, frequently seen in shock, may be caused by**

A an increased pulmonary capillary permeability
B cardiac failure
C fluid overload
D a reduced minute volume
E muscular weakness resulting in poor respiratory movement

17 A **False** This definition is incomplete. It does not include shock due to plasma or water loss, cardiogenic causes or shock which accompanies generalised septicaemia.
    B **True** This is the most comprehensive definition.
    C **False** Early bacteraemic shock is often characterised by warm extremities.
    D **False** This lay use of the term is irrelevant in the clinical situation.
    E **False** In septic shock cardiac output may be normal or high, but vasodilation results in poor tissue perfusion.

18 A **True** This is present in all forms of shock.
    B **False** The cardiac output is raised in early septicaemic shock.
    C **True** This is a comprehensive definition of the syndrome.
    D **False** In cases of cardiogenic shock the CVP is usually elevated.
    E **True** Poor tissue perfusion results in lactic acidosis and a lowered blood pH.

19 A **True** No single cause of the shock lung has been identified.
    B **True** Increased pulmonary permeability and cardiac failure together with fat embolism, oxygen toxicity and
    C **True** multiple microemboli in the pulmonary vessels may play a part. The frequent finding of pulmonary oedema in the absence of a raised central venous pressure or a decreased serum albumin, suggests that increased capillary permeability is the major cause. In cardiogenic shock and late hypovolaemia, cardiac failure plays a part. Fluid overload may occur and produce pulmonary oedema without right heart failure.
    D **False** The patient is usually hyperventilating and the minute volume is increased.
    E **False** Diminished respiratory effort does not usually play a part.

20 Important and urgent measures in the diagnosis and treatment of shock are

  A   warming the patient
  B   measurement of the central venous pressure
  C   noting the response of the central venous pressure to a rapid infusion of 200 to 500 ml of fluid
  D   urinary catheterisation
  E   arterial blood gas estimations

21 The metabolic acidosis of shock can be effectively treated by

  A   warming the patient
  B   administering sodium bicarbonate
  C   artificial ventilation
  D   restoring normal tissue perfusion
  E   intravenous infusions sufficient to maintain a normal central venous pressure (CVP)

22 In hypovolaemic shock

  A   the central venous pressure is low
  B   the difference in arteriovenous oxygen tension is unaffected
  C   the extremities are pale, cold and sweating
  D   urine output is unaffected
  E   there is always a site of bleeding

20 A **False** Although the skin vessels are usually contracted and the extremities cold this should be recognised as an effect rather than the cause of shock. Effective treatment will restore normal circulation.
    B **True**   It is important to ensure that the right atrial filling
    C **True**   pressure is sufficient to produce a normal cardiac
    D **True**   output. The response of the central venous pressure to a rapid fluid infusion is often necessary to distinguish cardiogenic from other forms of shock and normally the hourly urine volume will drop below 50 ml/hour when inadequate tissue perfusion is present.
    E **False** Blood gas estimations, though useful in monitoring effectiveness of treatment, have little part to play in the early management of shock.

21 A **False** The basic cause of the acidosis is poor tissue
    B **True**   perfusion and unless this is corrected there can be no
    C **False** permanent improvement. Bicarbonate is only necessary in cases of severe acidosis when a pH of below 7.1 may lead to serious cardiac arrhythmias.
    D **True**   Acidosis is a consequence of poor tissue perfusion.
    E **True**   The CVP provides the best guide as to whether adequate tissue perfusion is being achieved.

22 A **True**   This is due to the low circulating fluid volume.
    B **False** The associated decreased cardiac output leads to an increased arteriovenous difference in oxygen tension.
    C **True**   This is due to reflex sympathetic stimulae.
    D **False** The hourly urine volume falls because of decreased renal perfusion. Treatment should aim to maintain urine outflow at about 50 ml/hour.
    E **False** Hypovolaemia results not only from blood loss but from abnormal fluid loss or fluid sequestration in the tissues.

23 Hypovolaemic shock may result from

  A a 25 per cent third degree burn
  B generalised peritonitis
  C massive pulmonary embolism
  D intestinal obstruction
  E gastric outlet obstruction

24 Appropriate *immediate* intravenous infusions in all cases of non-cardiogenic shock are

  A whole blood
  B Ringer's lactate
  C normal saline
  D low molecular weight dextran
  E intravenous colloid solutions

25 Septic shock

  A is only caused by Gram-negative organisms
  B carries a favourable prognosis
  C produces a cellular defect that inhibits oxygen utilisation
  D is particularly associated with infective complications of the gastrointestinal and genitourinary systems
  E can be most effectively treated by antibiotics

23 A **True**   This is due to excessive sequestration of fluid in the
burned area and to serum losses.
   B **True**   This is due to fluid sequestration in the inflamed
peritoneum and adynamic bowel.
   C **False**   There is no change in the extracellular volume in this
condition although cardiogenic shock frequently
follows the reduced cardiac output.
   D **True**   Hypovolaemia results from excessive fluid loss due
to fluid sequestration in the distended bowel.
   E **True**   Decreased intake and loss due to vomiting result in
hypovolaemia.

24 A **False**   This should be restricted to cases of blood loss.
   B **True**   Both of these isotonic fluids satisfactorily expand the
   C **True**   plasma volume. The serum electrolytes should be
estimated as soon as possible to assess the long
term requirements. The haematocrit should be
checked to asess the need for blood.
   D **False**   This fluid has few advantages over Ringer's lactate or
saline and can produce spontaneous bleeding and
crossmatching problems.
   E **True**   Colloids such as hydroxymethyl starch or gelatin are
now widely used. They can produce adequate
resuscitation and produce few crossmatching or
anaphylactic problems.

25 A **False**   Although the commonest organisms are Gram-
negative, Gram-positive organisms and fungi may
also cause septic shock.
   B **False**   The mortality usually exceeds 30 per cent.
   C **True**   This may precede the haemodynamic changes.
   D **True**   This incidence is further increased by instrumental or
surgical manipulation of the infected region.
   E **False**   Endotoxins are the usual cause when septic shock is
manifest. Though antibiotics should be given they
can do nothing to counteract the endotoxins already
circulating.

26   Septic shock is particularly associated with
   A   thoracic surgical patients
   B   hypovolaemia
   C   indwelling urinary or intravenous catheters
   D   Gram-negative bacteraemia
   E   intra-abdominal sepsis

27   Septic shock is associated with a hypodynamic cardiovascular state
   A   if preceded by existing hypovolaemia
   B   in generalised peritonitis
   C   in mesenteric ischaemia
   D   when there is a Gram-positive bacteraemia
   E   in elderly patients

28   The diminished oxygen consumption in patients with septic shock is due to
   A   failure of oxygen transport in the lungs
   B   diminished blood flow in the periphery
   C   arteriovenous shunting in the periphery
   D   diminished oxygen utilisation by the cells
   E   diminished cardiac output

29   The mortality from septic shock can be effectively reduced by
   A   surgical drainage of abscesses
   B   the administration of appropriate antibiotics
   C   the restoration of a normal cardiovascular state
   D   positive pressure respiration
   E   the administration of H_2 antagonists

26 A **False** Both medical and surgical patients are at risk,
   B **True**   particularly those with hypovolaemia, septic foci and
   C **True**   indwelling intravenous cannulae or urinary catheters.
   D **True**   30 per cent of patients with a Gram-negative
              bacteraemia develop septic shock and this is
              commoner in patients with widespread neoplasia
              and in patients over the age of 50 years.
   E **True**   Gastrointestinal, renal and gynaecological infections
              caused by Gram-negative organisms are liable to
              produce this complication.

27 A **True**   In all cases where sepsis complicates a process
   B **True**   producing a loss of extracellular fluid volume such as
   C **True**   peritonitis, gangrenous bowel and intestinal
              obstruction, the hypodynamic pattern of shock is
              seen with a low central venous pressure, low cardiac
              output and cold sweaty extremities.
   D **False** This form of septic shock characteristically produces
              a hyperdynamic state.
   E **True**   These patients are particularly prone to septic shock.

28 A **True**   The pulmonary oedema associated with septic shock
              impairs oxygen uptake.
   B **False** Even in hyperdynamic states, where peripheral blood
              flow is increased, there is a deficient oxygen uptake
              due to impaired cellular functions.
   C **False** Xenon clearance studies have not shown any
              peripheral arteriovenous shunting in these patients.
   D **True**   Vital cell functions are impaired with a resultant
              inability to utilise oxygen.
   E **True**   This is almost invariably present.

29 A **True**   Patients have a better prognosis after drainage.
   B **True**   The mortality rate is halved when effective antibiotics
              are used.
   C **True**   This may require blood or saline infusions and
              possibly the administration of isoprenaline
              dobutamine and digitalis.
   D **True**   Mechanical ventilation should not be restricted to
              those patients with specific respiratory indications.
   E **True**   Stress ulceration of the gastrointestinal tract is very
              common in these patients. The incidence can be
              diminished by the use of H_2 blockade.

30 In cardiogenic shock
   A the central venous pressure is low
   B the difference in the arteriovenous oxygen tension is increased
   C the haemotocrit is raised
   D the blood pressure is unaffected
   E urinary flow rates are unchanged

31 Prospective blood donors
   A should be asked about previous attacks of jaundice
   B should be asked about recent travel itinerary
   C should have serological tests for syphilis
   D may transmit glandular fever to a recipient
   E may transmit malaria to a recipient

32 A blood transfusion reaction
   A may be due to incompatibility of the recipient serum and donor cells
   B is manifest by thrombophlebitis of the infusion site
   C occurs within the first 30 minutes of transfusion
   D may produce renal damage
   E must be suspected when the patient complains of loin pain

30 A **False**   There is usually an increased central venous
                    pressure.
    B **True**   This is due to inadequate tissue perfusion.
    C **False**   The haematocrit is unchanged whereas in
                    hypovolaemic shock not due to blood loss it is raised.
    D **False**   The inadequate cardiac output always produces a fall
    E **False**   in blood pressure and hourly urine production falls.

31 A **True**   Donors who have had serum or infective hepatitis
                    may remain infective for up to 3 years. A few become
                    carriers.
    B **True**   The risk of HIV infection is feared. Prospective donors
                    who have recently travelled in the Third World where
                    HIV is more common are now not accepted as blood
                    transfusion donors in many countries. In the UK
                    there is an additional safety precaution; all potential
                    donors are tested for HIV.
    C **True**   Spirochaetes are transmissible (they will survive for 4
                    days in stored blood). Gonorrhoea is not
                    transmissible.
    D **True**   This infection is transmissible.
    E **True**   In some countries malarial donors are not accepted
                    although the serum alone may be used without risk
                    of transmission.

32 A **True**   Mismatching produces agglutination of the donor
                    cells.
    B **False**   The signs include fever, chills, breathlessness and
                    pain in the flanks and chest. These may be followed
                    by hypotension, haemorrhagic phenomena and
                    haemoglobinuria.
    C **True**   This period should be closely observed when a blood
                    transfusion is commenced.
    D **True**   This is the result of haemoglobinuria, hypotension
    E **True**   and acidosis. Renal pain is a frequent manifestation.
                    It should be treated by immediately stopping the
                    transfusion, invoking a diuresis and restoring the
                    patient's blood pressure.

33   Pyrexial reactions to blood transfusions
   A   have increased since the introduction of sterile disposable
         infusion sets
   B   may be caused by allergic reactions
   C   may be caused by contaminated blood
   D   may be a response to a large blood transfusion
   E   should be treated by stopping the transfusion

34   Massive blood transfusions may be complicated by
   A   hyperkalaemia
   B   hypercalcaemia
   C   hepatic coma
   D   leucopenia
   E   coagulopathy

33 A **False** Pyrogen reactions have decreased since the
introduction of disposable infusion sets.
    B **True**   This is due to allergens in the donor blood.
    C **True**   Gram-negative endotoxins are the commonest cause
and bacteria may multiply in warm blood. Blood
should therefore be stored at 4°C until it is required.
    D **False** This produces a fall in body temperature.
    E **True**   The transfusion must be stopped since some of the
causes are potentially fatal.

34 A **True**   In 3-week-old blood the plasma potassium rises to 30
to 40 mEq (30 to 40 mmol)/litre.
    B **False** Hypocalcaemia may occur and this is accentuated if
citrate is used as the anticoagulant. It should be
treated by the administration of calcium chloride.
    C **True**   This may occur in cirrhotic patients, possibly due to a
high ammonia concentration.
    D **False** There is no change in the white cell count.
    E **True**   Donated blood is usually low in platelets.
Coagulation problems may respond to fresh frozen
plasma.

3 Burns

35 When determining the depth of a burn
A a knowledge of the type of injury is important
B the presence of blisters is of no clinical significance
C impairment of sensibility of the burned area should be tested
D the presence of severe pain denotes a full thickness skin loss
E assessment within the first 24 hours is essential to the planning of treatment

36 Estimation of the area of a burn
A is of very little clinical significance
B when extensive, is best undertaken after the patient has been resuscitated
C provides important prognostic information
D is an important factor in the estimation of the fluid required
E can be based on a formula which states that the adult trunk is 36 per cent of the whole body surface area

37 Patients with major burns
A are in a negative nitrogen balance
B have normal calorie requirements
C do not generally become anaemic
D are resistant to septicaemia
E may suffer gastrointestinal complications

35 A **True** Contact with hot liquids usually causes partial thickness loss, whereas flames commonly give rise to full thickness losses.

B **False** Blisters do not occur in full thickness loss.

C **True** Full thickness burns have a reduced pain sensibility.

D **False** Nerve endings in the area of a full thickness burn are usually destroyed.

E **False** During this period resuscitation and prevention of infection are the predominant aims. Depth of burn and its consequences can usually be assessed later.

36 A **False** The form of therapy and the fluid requirements of the patient are determined by the area of the burn.

B **False** The area determines the fluid requirement and is a necessary urgent assessment.

C **True** The prognosis after a burn injury is related to the extent of the burn.

D **True** This is an important guide, although no formula for fluid therapy in burns can be precise. It is also important to carefully monitor indices of tissue perfusion and cardiovascular status, such as hourly urine volume and ventral venous pressure measurements.

E **True** In the adult, the 'Rule of Nines', wherein the head and upper limbs each measure 9 per cent and the lower limbs 18 per cent each, is widely used as a rough guide in estimating the area of a burn.

37 A **True** Even if the greatly increased needs of 150 to 200 g protein/day are met the negative nitrogen balance will persist until the wound is healed.

B **False** Calorie requirements may be at least twice normal due to increased energy losses through increased evaporative water loss and fever. Nutritional supplements are thus frequently necessary.

C **False** There is blood destruction and sequestration in the early days of a burn. These factors together with infection and septicaemia give rise to anaemia.

D **False** They have an increased susceptibility to infection and have many more potential sources of infection than a healthy patient.

E **True** 'Stress' ulceration of the stomach and duodenum may complicate major burns.

38 The catabolic response to trauma and infection
   A   results in an increase in lean body mass
   B   results in a positive nitrogen balance
   C   results in gluconeogenesis
   D   causes a falling haemoglobin level
   E   is mediated by the adrenals

39 The catabolic response to trauma
   A   is related to the severity of the trauma
   B   is accompanied by increased urinary losses of potassium
       and nitrogen
   C   can be prevented by parenteral nutrition
   D   does not occur in the adrenalectomised patient
   E   helps to increase muscular power tone in the traumatised
       patient

40 Fluid losses in a major burn are
   A   maximal between 12 and 24 hours after the injury
   B   related to the age of the patient
   C   related to the weight of the patient
   D   related to the area burnt
   E   are most significant in burns of the limbs

38 A **False**   A breakdown of tissue protein provides substrates
    B **False**   for gluconeogenesis. There is thus a loss of most
    C **True**   body tissue proteins, this being reflected by a
                    decrease of the lean body mass and a negative
                    nitrogen balance.
    D **False**   Haemoglobin synthesis is usually unaffected in the
                    catabolic phase.
    E **True**   The response is initiated by catecholamines released
                    from the adrenals.

39 A **True**   Whereas a patient with a fractured femur will lose
                    approximately 11 g of nitrogen (70 g of protein)/day,
                    a major burn may lose 40 g of nitrogen/day.
    B **True**   Following protein catabolism and gluconeogenesis.
    C **False**   Parentally administered amino acids, when suitably
                    admixed with a source of calories, minimise but do
                    not abolish the catabolic response.
    D **False**   There is no known dependence on the endocrine
                    system.
    E **False**   Catabolism results in gluconeogenesis: protein,
                    whose major source is skeletal muscle, is
                    metabolised to produce energy.

40 A **False**   They are maximal in the first 8 hours after burning.
    B **False**   There is no known relationship to age but there is a
    C **True**   direct relationship to body weight, the area burnt and
    D **True**   the depth of the burn. Many guides to fluid therapy in
                    the burned patient take account of these factors, e.g.:
                        First 24 hours:
                            (i) electrolyte solution 1.5 ml/kg/per cent body
                                 surface burn
                            (ii) colloid solution 0.5 ml/kg/per cent body
                                 surface burn.
                        Plus metabolic requirements (approximately 2000
                        ml in an adult). Half the above fluid is given
                        intravenously in the first 8 hours and one-quarter in
                        each of the succesive 8 hours.
    E **False**   The amount of skin burnt rather than its situation
                    determines the fluid losses expected.

41 The increased fluid requirements of a patient with a full thickness burn are due to

A   increased evaporative water loss
B   sequestration of fluid in the injured tissues
C   inflammatory pneumonia
D   serum exuding from the burned area
E   destruction of blood in the skin vessels

42 48 hours after a major burn and with satisfactory fluid therapy a patient

A   has very few abnormal fluid losses
B   may need a blood transfusion
C   is often hypernatraemic
D   usually needs skin grafting
E   requires prophylactic antibiotics

43 Major burns are sometimes complicated by

A   acute gastric and duodenal ulcers
B   paralytic ileus
C   cerebral oedema
D   mesenteric thrombosis
E   septicaemia

41 A **True**   Evaporative water loss from a full thickness burn is
    B **True**   more than 10 times that of intact skin. Two and a half
    C **True**   litres of water may be lost per day from a 40 per cent
    D **True**   burn. There is a local (and to a lesser extent, a
                  general) increase in capillary permeability so that
                  protein-rich fluid gains the interstitial space from the
                  blood. Large amounts of fluid are sequestrated in the
                  inflammation which surrounds the burn injury.
                  Relatively little serum is lost from a full thickness
                  burn.
    E **False** Although there is some destruction of red cells and a
                  diminution in the red cell mass this is not an
                  important factor in accounting for the increased fluid
                  requirements.

42 A **False** Insensible evaporative water loss is still excessive –
                  up to 3 litres/day in the adult with extensive burns.
    B **True**   Destruction of red cells, trapping of blood in
                  thrombosed capillaries and increased phagocytosis
                  of red cells may produce anaemia at this time.
    C **True**   This is mainly due to increased insensible losses of
                  water
    D **False** Surgical debridement of a major burn at this time is
                  very traumatic and is rarely indicated. Skin grafting is
                  sometimes undertaken after 7 days but there is a
                  need for great care in limiting the blood loss if
                  surgical removal of the eschar is undertaken.
    E **True**   Penicillin is often employed because streptococci
                  frequently colonise burned areas.

43 A **True**   The ulcers are known as Curling's ulcers. They are
                  frequently multiple in the stomach and most
                  common in extensive burns.
    B **True**   This often lasts 48 to 72 hours.
    C **True**   This is maximal 48 to 72 hours after the injury when
                  the risk of hyponatraemia due to over transfusion
                  with intravenous fluids is greatest.
    D **False** There is no recognised relationship.
    E **True**   The burned area is a gigantic portal for infections and
                  septicaemia is common.

44   In a burned patient, associated pulmonary injury
   A   should be suspected in head and neck burns
   B   should be suspected when the nasal hairs are burnt
   C   does not appear clinically in the first 24 hours
   D   may be avoided by the prophylactic use of antibiotics
   E   may result in pneumonia

45   Secondary infection of burns is
   A   less common in partial than in full thickness skin loss
   B   relatively more common in burns of more than 20 per cent
       body area
   C   avoided by leaving the burn eschar intact
   D   avoided by the immediate application of a sterile occlusive
       dressing
   E   prevented by antibiotic prophylaxis

46   Scalds
   A   are more frequent in children
   B   commonly cause full thickness skin loss
   C   should be skin grafted within 48 hours of the injury
   D   need routine antibiotic treatment
   E   can have their consequences minimised by cold water
       immersion

47   The dressing of a small burn should be
   A   occlusive
   B   non-absorptive
   C   non-compressive
   D   changed daily as a routine
   E   avoided so that an eschar can form

44 A **True**   The additional sign of pharyngeal inflammation may
    B **True**   be present and should be looked for.
    C **False**   The effects of burn injury to the lungs are often
                    immediate.
    D **False**   Antibiotics do not prevent the injury but may prevent
                    secondary infection.
    E **True**   Inhalation of burning gases produces much
                    pulmonary inflammation and subsequent pneumonia
                    is common.

45 A **True**   The protective function of the skin against invasive
    B **False**   infection by environmental organisms is lost when a
                    full thickness burn is present. To a large extent this
                    protective function is retained in a partial thickness
                    burn. Small burns are as readily infected as large
                    burns.
    C **False**   The dry dead burn eschar is permeable and is an
                    entry site for invasive infection.
    D **False**   Viable bacteria may remain in the follicles deep to
                    the burned surface and subsequently multiply to
                    infect the area.
    E **True**   Providing they are administered at the outset.

46 A **True**   This is especially so in children under 3 years of age.
    B **False**   Hot or boiling water usually produces partial skin
                    loss.
    C **False**   Local cleansing and the application of a non-adherent
    D **False**   sterile dressing are all that is usually required.
                    Healing generally takes place uneventfully without
                    the need for grafting or antibiotic therapy.
    E **True**   Immediate immersion in cold water is the most
                    effective act a 'first aider' can perform. Tissue
                    damage is in this way limited.

47 A **True**   The aim of the dressing is to prevent bacterial
    B **False**   invasion and to provide firm compression and
    C **False**   support. If these criteria are met, it need only be
    D **False**   changed every 4 or 5 days. The infected burn will
                    require dressing daily or more frequently.
    E **False**   Absence of dressing renders infection more likely
                    and the resulting fibrosis will diminish the eventual
                    functional result.

48   A partial thickness burn

A   may heal without grafting
B   may deteriorate into full thickness skin loss
C   rarely causes severe physiological derangement of the patient
D   heals within 7 days in the absence of infection
E   can be diagnosed clinically

49   The early management of a burn wound may include

A   early excision
B   occlusive dressings
C   exposure treatment
D   dressings with local antibiotics
E   skin grafting

50   Skin grafting of a full thickness burn wound

A   should usually be with full thickness skin grafts
B   is more likely to be successful if undertaken in the first week after injury
C   will be unsuccessful unless the wound surface is sterile
D   minimises scar contracture
E   is rarely essential

48 A **True**   Epithelial regeneration will spread from the epithelial remnants in the hair follicles and deeper layers of the epidermis.
    B **True**   Infection may convert it into a full thickness skin loss by destroying the remaining dermal elements.
    C **False** In a deep partial thickness burn there is a considerable inflammatory response even though some epidermal elements may have escaped injury. If the burn is of more than 15 to 20 per cent of the body surface, hypovolaemia may develop.
    D **False** The deeper partial thickness burns may require 3 or 4 weeks before epithelial regeneration is complete.
    E **True**   Blistering and preservation of the deep dermal elements, so that epithelial regeneration can be seen occurring around the separate islands of the hair follicles, facilitate the diagnosis of partial thickness burn.

49 A **True**   All these treatments are acceptable depending on the
    B **True**   type of burns; minor partial thickness burns may
    C **True**   warrant outpatient management with occlusive
    D **True**   dressings and small full thickness burns early excision. In major burns, fluid therapy has priority and the burn is treated as the circumstances dictate.
    E **True**   Partial thickness skin grafting should be employed once the granulating skin wound is clean.

50 A **False** With the exception of very small burns of the eyelids or the delayed treatment of contractures (when full thickness pedicle grafts may be used), split thickness skin grafts are used.
    B **False** Grafting is less successful before granulation tissue is present. However homo- or heterograft skin may be used as a very effective burn dressing in the early stages of repair.
    C **False** Although beta-haemolytic streptococci are inimical to skin grafts, moderate infections of the wounds with other organisms are not a contraindication of skin grafting.
    D **True**   For this reason burns around joints should receive early attention.
    E **False** Skin grafting reduces the subsequent contractions of the burn wound.

4 Wound healing, surgical infection and postoperative complications

51 A clean incised skin wound

- A undergoes an inflammatory phase during the processes of repair
- B commences epithelialisation after 7 to 10 days
- C regains the full strength of normal skin within 10 days
- D regains its strength as the result of fibroblast activity
- E does not undergo contraction

52 Wound healing is

- A impaired in anaemic patients
- B impaired by haematoma formation
- C impaired by hypoproteinaemia
- D stimulated by steroids
- E more rapid in the young than in the old

51 A **True** Polymorphs and monocytes accumulate and engulf cell debris and all foreign material during the initial phase of repair.

B **False** A clean incised wound whose edges are opposed is re-epithelialised within 2 days.

C **False** A healed skin wound is never as strong as unwounded skin. After 8 weeks it has reached 80 per cent of its original strength.

D **True** These cells synthesise collagen.

E **False** All wounds contract and do so from end to end. This is thought to be brought about by myofibroblasts within the granulation tissue.

---

52 A **False** No studies have confirmed this widely held view.

B **True** Any foreign material, fluid or haematoma prolongs the inflammatory phase and inhibits fibroblast invasion.

C **True** An albumin concentration below 2.5 g/100 ml significantly impairs wound healing.

D **False** Steroids decrease the rate of epithelialisation and inhibit fibroblast proliferation. They thus have an inhibitory effect on wound healing.

E **True** The fibroblastic response and cellular proliferation are more rapid in the young.

53 The principles of wound care include
  A early skin cover
  B removal of foreign material
  C routine administration of antibiotics
  D layered apposition of uninfected wounded tissues
  E routine use of drains

54 Heavily contaminated and dirty wounds
  A require surgical toilet and delayed closure
  B require the administration of systemic antibiotics
  C can usually be treated by wound toilet and primary closure
  D should be totally excised
  E should be allowed to heal by secondary intention and possible skin grafting

55 Surgical drainage of abscesses
  A should be via a small incision with minimal disturbance of the adjacent tissues
  B should be dependent wherever possible
  C has been outmoded by antibiotic therapy
  D should be undertaken before the signs of fluctuation appear
  E should not be continued for more than 48 hours

53 A **True**   The principles of meticulous debridement and careful
    B **True**   tissue apposition should be adhered to whether the
    C **False** wound is from a sterile surgical knife or is the untidy
    D **True**   contaminated wound of a road traffic accident. Skin
               grafts should cover skin defects as soon as possible.
               When wound toilet is not possible within 12 to 18
               hours it is usually best to delay closure of the wound
               because by this time active bacterial multiplication
               has occurred. Antibiotics should only be used when
               infection is likely to have occurred.
    E **False** Drains have no place in the care of clean tidy
               wounds. If there is doubt about presence of infection
               or foreign material the wound should be left open.

54 A **True**   Meticulous removal of dead and foreign material
    B **True**   coupled with the administration of a suitable broad
    C **False** spectrum antibiotic and gentle packing with gauze
               prior to delayed closure 4 or 5 days later is the most
               effective form of treatment.
    D **False** The remaining wound would be scarcely less
               contaminated and such radical therapy is usually
               only necessary in spreading infections such as gas
               gangrene.
    E **False** Healing by delayed primary closure will produce
               better functional results than the scarring and wound
               contractions that would follow this very conservative
               course of management.

55 A **False** Bold incisions, with the breaking down of all loculi
               and the removal of slough, should be undertaken.
    B **True**   Gravity will help drainage.
    C **False** Antibiotics are of little value in the treatment of an
               abscess but, when cellulitis surrounds the abscess,
               they should be used as an adjunct to surgery.
    D **False** At this point the infection may be at the cellulitic
               stage and not localised. It is then justifiable to
               administer antibiotics and carefully observe the
               response. (Fluctuation is, of course, only elicited in
               palpable abscesses.)
    E **False** Drainage of a collection of pus is therapeutic but only
               if it is continued for as long as there is material to
               discharge.

56   In localised surgical infections
   A   an elevated leucocyte count is usually present
   B   fever and tenderness are usually present
   C   the presence of glycosuria usually indicates metastatic
         pancreatic abscesses.
   D   pus is frequently absent
   E   pain is always a prominent symptom

57   Staphylococcal infections
   A   do not cause cellulitis
   B   do not produce septicaemia
   C   do not produce fever
   D   produce yellow odourless pus
   E   may be airborne infections

58   Streptococcal infections
   A   are characterised by abscess formation
   B   rarely produce lymphadenitis
   C   frequently produce bacteraemia
   D   can produce a gangrenous skin infection
   E   can be treated by antibiotics without surgical intervention

56 A **True**   But in an infection attenuated by prolonged and only
    B **True**   partially effective antibiotic therapy these common
               signs are frequently absent.
    C **False** Diabetes and infection do however frequently co-
               exist and make the treatment of each more difficult.
               Pancreatic abscesses are not associated with
               diabetes.
    D **False** It is a characteristic of all localised infections that pus
               (necrotic cellular debris, macrophages and bacteria)
               is found surrounded by granulation tissue and
               fibrosis (the abscess wall).
    E **False** When abscesses are attenuated by antibiotic therapy
               or develop in situations where they are not confined,
               such as in the subphrenic spaces, pain does not
               occur.

---

57 A **False** Staphylococcal cellulitis does occur.
    B **False** Septicaemia does occur and may be accompanied by
               septic shock and metastatic abscess formation.
    C **False** Pyrexia is present in all but the smallest skin
               eruptions.
    D **True**   This characterises a staphylococcal abscess.
    E **True**   Most airborne staphylococci are carried on skin
               squames, contaminated from the nose.
               Staphylococcal skin lesions disperse the bacteria
               even more heavily.

---

58 A **False** They are characteristically invasive and produce
               cellulitis.
    B **False** Lymphangitis and lymphadenitis are common.
    C **True**   This should be suspected when pyrexia, rigor or
               toxaemia develops.
    D **True**   Streptococcal gangrene, due to anaerobic organisms,
               is characterised by oedema and haemorrhagic skin
               bullae. It may be confused with a clostridial cellulitis.
    E **True**   Fibrosis and abscess formation rarely occur. The
               appropriate antibiotics are often successful in
               treating these infections.

59 Tetanus prophylaxis in a patient with a badly contaminated wound
  A depends, even in an actively immunised patient, on meticulous immediate debridement of the wound
  B should include the administration of tetanus toxoid
  C is more safely achieved with equine rather than human antitoxin
  D is unnecessary in patients who have been recently actively immunised
  E should include antibiotic therapy

60 Tetanus
  A may have an incubation period of over 20 days
  B can be prevented by the immediate administration of tetanus toxoid
  C is more common after scalp lacerations than wounds of the extremities
  D is usually associated with stupor or coma
  E is always associated with an injury

61 The treatment of established tetanus
  A should include wound excision
  B has been improved by the use of mechanical ventilation
  C requires adequate and prolonged antibiotic therapy
  D should include treatment with human antitetanus antitoxin
  E is more successful when the disease has a short onset

59 A **True** This is *essential* and cannot be over-emphasised.
    B **True** The previously unimmunised patient should also receive antitetanus toxin; the actively immunised patient requires a booster dose or toxoid.
    C **False** The antibody titre remains higher for a longer period with the human antitoxin. The equine variety is complicated by allergic reactions and cross-sensitivity in about half the patients.
    D **False** See B – prophylaxis should *always* include wound care.
    E **True** Penicillin should be given together with wound cleansing and debridement.

60 A **True** This may vary from 3 to 24 days.
    B **False** Active immunisation will not confer protection for 2 to 3 weeks after the injection of the toxoid. Wounds which are contaminated with foreign bodies or necrotic tissue are particularly at risk. Prophylaxis should include adequate wound toilet and passive immunisation of the previously unimmunised patient. Patients who have had a full course of active immunisation with toxoid require a booster dose.
    C **False** Injuries of the extremities are more frequently compliated by tetanus. The rich blood supply of the scalp confers some protection.
    D **False** The patient's conscious level is rarely depressed.
    E **False** Under 60 per cent of cases have a known injury. In others, the source of the toxin may be infection of an area of broken skin or a surgical wound. In many cases the injury is so trivial that it passes undetected.

61 A **True** This will prevent the release of further exotoxins.
    B **True** The spasms and clonic contractions that characterise the severe infection are painful, distressing and may interfere with respiration. Thus, these cases may need treatment with muscle relaxants, sedatives and mechanical ventilation.
    C **False** Although antibiotics may be required for the initial treatment of the causative wound, they are ineffective in the treatment of established tetanus whose effects are caused by toxins.
    D **True** The human, rather than the equine, antitoxin allows successive doses of antitoxin to be given subcutaneously and systematically. It has improved the results of treatment.
    E **False** The disease is frequently more severe and has a worse outcome when the incubation period is short.

62 Clostridial myositis

    A   is otherwise known as gas gangrene
    B   has a 2 to 3 week incubation period
    C   may produce jaundice
    D   may rapidly produce anaemia
    E   requires early treatment with antitoxins

63 In clostridial infections

    A   a spreading cellulitis may be present
    B   Gram-positive cocci can be isolated from the discharge
    C   surgical treatment has a minor part to play
    D   gas production is often absent
    E   thrombosis contributes to the clinical picture

64 Actinomyosis is characterised by

    A   chronic abscesses of the cervicofacial region
    B   a granulomatous abscess wall
    C   red coloured pus
    D   a palpable, tender inflammatory mass
    E   its resistance to antibiotics

62　A　**True**　It is caused most frequently by *Clostridium perfringens (welchii)* and *septicum.*
　　B　**False**　This is a very rapidly progressive infection generally associated with a poor blood supply and delayed surgical care to contaminated wounds.
　　C　**True**　The many clostridial exotoxins giving rise to severe
　　D　**True**　systemic effects include potent haemolysins.
　　E　**False**　Antitoxins have only a limited value. Excisional surgery, penicillin and supportive measures are more appropriate.

63　A　**True**　*Clostridium perfringens (welchii)* may cause this serious condition. It is characterised by a rapidly spreading crepitant cellulitis.
　　B　**False**　Clostridia are Gram-positive rod shaped bacilli.
　　C　**False**　Early desloughing, wound toilet and surgical decompression by incision and fasciotomy are essential. Antibiotics are an adjunct to surgery.
　　D　**True**　*Clostridium tetani* does not generally produce gas and gas production in *Clostridium perfringens (welchii)* cellulitis and myositis may be absent. Streptococcal cellulitis and mixed infections sometimes produce gas in the tissues.
　　E　**True**　Endothelial damage from the toxins results in thrombosis which further contributes to tissue necrosis.

64　A　**True**　Other common sites are the chest wall and the caecum.
　　B　**True**　The fibrotic abscess wall contains many granulomas
　　C　**False**　and tangled masses of branching filaments ('sulphur' granules) which give a characteristic yellow colour to the pus.
　　D　**True**　A tender mass usually results.
　　E　**False**　The infection can be effectively treated by a 3 to 4 week course of penicillin or tetracycline.

65   A subphrenic abscess
  A   is usually accompanied by considerable systemic effects
  B   is associated with local rib tenderness
  C   rarely produces abnormal signs in the chest
  D   may be diagnosed by a barium meal examination
  E   may be best diagnosed by an ultrasound scan

66   A pelvic abscess
  A   lies extraperitoneally
  B   may be a complication of abdominal surgery
  C   often presents with diarrhoea
  D   can be readily diagnosed by clinical examination
  E   should be treated with antibiotics alone

65 A **False** The signs and symptoms of this condition are frequently minimal, with only a mild pyrexia and a leucocytosis being present.

B **True** Occasionally there is tenderness between the

C **False** overlying ribs, a sympathetic pleural effusion in the adjacent pleural cavity, shoulder tip pain and hiccoughs.

D **True** A left-sided subphrenic abscess may be noted on barium meal by indentation of the fundus of the stomach. Diminished diaphragmatic movement may be observed fluoroscopically.

E **True** Ultrasound scans have largely replaced fluoroscopic techniques, as they are simple and noninvasive, and provide accurate localisation for percutaneous drainage.

66 A **False** This abscess lies in the lowest cul-de-sac of peritoneum, the rectovesical or recto-uterine pouch.

B **True** It may also result from an infected neighbouring viscus, e.g. appendix or from generalised peritonitis.

C **True** Watery diarrhoea frequently results from associated rectal inflammation. The systemic effects of an abscess are also present.

D **True** Most abscesses are palpable as a tender pelvic mass, lying anterior to the rectum.

E **False** Antibiotics are useful when the pelvic infection is at the cellulitic stage and as an adjunct to surgery. They cannot alone treat an established abscess and drainage is required. Drainage is most readily effected through the anterior rectal wall, once the abscess has been confirmed by needle aspiration.

67 Paralytic ileus
A is associated with electrolyte imbalance
B may be associated with mechanical intestinal obstruction
C requires treatment with nasogastric suction and intravenous fluids
D is associated with retroperitoneal haematoma
E will sometimes respond to atropine

68 Acute postoperative gastric dilatation
A may cause postoperative vascular collapse
B can be prevented by regular nasogastric aspiration
C characteristically occurs on the first postoperative day
D is a relatively common problem after surgery on the gastrointestinal tract
E is not a dangerous or threatening complication

69 The appearance of jaundice in the postoperative period
A may indicate an intraperitoneal haemorrhage
B is usually due to the toxic effects of anaesthetic agents
C may be due to septicaemia
D may indicate chronic liver disease
E may well result in delayed wound healing

67 A **True**   There are abnormal fluid and electrolyte losses in a patient with paralytic ileus. Hypokalaemia particularly contributes to further inhibition of intestinal motility by interfering with the normal ionic movements during smooth muscle contraction.

   B **True**   Prolonged intestinal distension such as is associated with mechanical intestinal obstruction may also inhibit intestinal motility.

   C **True**   Decompression of the distended bowel by nasogastric suction and replacement of the abnormal fluid losses form the basis of treatment after mechanical causes of the obstruction have been ruled out.

   D **True**   Retroperitoneal haemorrhage, severe trauma, particularly to the vertebral column, and ureteric distension all inhibit intestinal motility.

   E **False**   Pharmacological treatment has not yet been shown to be effective.

68 A **True**   Gastric distention (with up to 5 or 6 litres of fluid) is associated with hypovolaemia.

   B **True**   This is frequently prescribed for the first 2 to 3 postoperative days until flatus is passed and bowel sounds return to normal.

   C **False**   It usually occurs 2 to 3 days after abdominal operations.

   D **False**   The routine use of postoperative nasogastric suction has almost abolished its incidence after abdominal surgery. It still occurs in severe injuries and burns where nasogastric suction is less commonly used.

   E **False**   Patients with this complication are at risk from profuse vomiting and aspiration of gastric contents.

69 A **True**   The blood is haemolysed producing a transient mild haemolytic jaundice.

   B **False**   Certain anaesthetic agents (such as chloroform and possibly halothane) have a hepatotoxic effect, but the incidence is very low.

   C **True**   Severe sepsis may give rise to jaundice, probably by haemolysis.

   D **True**   Hypotension and hypoxia during the operative period may precipitate jaundice in a patient with chronic liver disease.

   E **False**   Jaundice does not affect wound healing.

70   A small bowel fistula
A   loses intestinal fluid rich in potassium and sodium
B   may give rise to a metabolic acidosis
C   rapidly results in dehydration
D   usually results in skin excoriation
E   may be managed conservatively by the abandonment of oral feeding

71   A pancreatic fistula
A   loses fluids with higher potassium and lower sodium levels than plasma
B   may give rise to a metabolic acidosis
C   will usually close if oral feeding is temporarily suspended
D   may heal with somatostatin treatment
E   almost always requires surgical treatment

72   Bed sores
A   can be prevented by sheepskin blankets
B   can be prevented by changing the patient's position four times each 24 hours
C   are the consequence of local infection
D   only occur over the sacrum
E   may heal spontaneously

70 A **True** The concentration of sodium in the fistulous fluid is comparable to plasma and that of potassium often higher.

B **True** This is due to the alkaline nature of the fistulous losses.

C **True** Water losses may be as much as 4 or 5 litres per day.

D **True** The alkaline fistula fluid and some enzyme activity produce early skin excoriation.

E **True** Provided there is no distal obstruction, parenteral nutrition and the cessation of oral feeding may result in a decrease of the fistulous losses and eventual closure.

71 A **False** The sodium and potassium levels in pancreatic fluid are similar to those of plasma.

B **True** There are high bicarbonate losses.

C **False** The high concentration of enzymes renders skin excoriation a major problem and abandonment of oral feeding will only slightly diminish the volume of fistula losses. It thus has little effect on the healing of the fistula.

D **True** Somatostatin diminishes the volume of

E **False** pancreatic fluid and may effect a cure but if this is unsuccessful, due to major duct obstruction or damage, then surgery may be needed.

72 A **False** Bed sores are due to local ischaemia. This may occur

B **False** over any bony prominences, the back of the head,

C **False** the heels and the greater trochanter of the femur as

D **False** well as the sacrum. They are often the consequence of inadequate nursing (and medical) care and observation. They are best prevented by changing the patient's position every 2 hours. Sheepskin and foam underlays add support to the nursing endeavours but cannot alone prevent their development.

E **True** Most 'acute' pressure sores will heal spontaneously if careful wound care is given but chronic ulcers will need surgical help, by skin grafting or a musculocutaneous flap.

Skin and breast

73 Malignant melanomata
   A occur more commonly in the black races F
   B occur with equal frequency in all ages F
   C frequently arise from pre-existing benign naevi T
   D occur more frequently in tropical regions T
   E are commonest on the trunk F

74 A malignant melanoma
   A frequently arises from hair-bearing naevi F   Best pro[?]osis
   B frequently arises from junctional naevi T
   C has a worse prognosis when it arises on the leg T
   D should be suspected in any pigmented lesion which bleeds
      spontaneously T
   E may be invisible T

7/10

73 A **False** They are rare in the black races where they are usually found only in the depigmented skin of the feet and hands.
    B **False** They usually present between the ages of 30 and 60 years. They are very rare in the prepubertal child.
    C **True** Approximately half the patients give a history of change in a pre-existing stable pigmented lesion.
    D **True** The incidence in the white races is related quite closely to the amount of solar radiation received. The highest incidence is in white Australians.
    E **False** In Australia as elsewhere they are commonest on those parts of the skin most exposed to the sun.

74 A **False** These naevi contain dermal elements and have a very low malignant potential. _— hair_
    B **True** These flat, usually darkly pigmented lesions are _— junctional_ those most likely to undergo malignant change.
    C **False** Lower limb melanomata have the best prognosis. Head, neck and trunk melanomata have the worst. Late recognition is thought to be a factor in explaining the poor survival of the latter group.
    D **True** This is a warning sign, together with itching, ulceration, progressive growth and increased pigmentation.
    E **True** A small proportion present first with a metastasis, the primary being an amelanotic melanoma.

75 The treatment of a malignant melanoma should include
    A a preliminary incision biopsy
    B wide excision of the tumour
    C 'en bloc' removal of adjacent involved lymph nodes
    D immediate excision of any enlarging lymph node in the
       postoperative period
    E radiotherapy to the surgical area and adjacent lymph nodes

76 Squamous cancer of the lip
    A is most common in early adult life
    B is more common in fair skinned subjects
    C is more frequent in females
    D metastasises readily by the bloodstream
    E is preferably treated by radiotherapy once lymph node
       deposits are present

75 A **False**   Dissemination by blood and lymphatic systems
                   frequently follows this procedure.
    B **True**   The extent of the excision is related not only to the
                   size and site of the primary, but also to the type.
                   Protuberant lesions infiltrate surrounding lymphatics
                   radically and should be excised with 2 to 3 cm
                   margins. Flat lesions may be successfully treated
                   with a more limited excision.
    C **True**   But the policy regarding 'prophylactic' lymph node
                   removal, when they are remote from the tumour and
                   possibly uninvolved, is less certain and much
                   controversy exists.
    D **True**   Examinations should be carried out every 1 to 3
                   months for at least the first 2 years. Enlargement of
                   regional nodes is then noted early and is an
                   indication for immediate excision of those nodes. In
                   this way systemic spread can be avoided in some
                   patients.
    E **False**   Radiotherapy is ineffective, whether used
                   prophylactically or therapeutically.

76 A **False**   There is an increasing incidence with age. It is
    B **True**   common in people exposed to large amounts of
                   sunlight particularly if their skin has little natural
                   pigmentation. It is very rare in the black races.
    C **False**   Males are much more commonly affected.
    D **False**   The most common mode of spread is by direct
                   extension to neighbouring tissues. Lymphatic spread
                   does occur, particularly in poorly differentiated
                   lesions, but spread via the bloodstream is
                   uncommon.
    E **False**   Surgical excision is recommended with block
                   dissection of the neck if there is evidence of lymph
                   node metastasis. Radiotherapy on its own is
                   indicated for small well-differentiated lesions, when
                   the possibility of metastasis is unlikely, or as
                   palliative treatment in the late stages of the disease.

77 Basal cell carcinomas

A are commonest on the face and neck
B usually metastasise to regional lymph nodes
C are less common than squamous cell carcinomas
D are characterised histologically by epithelial pearls
E are particularly common in oriental races

78 Capillary angiomas of childhood (strawberry naevi)

A arise in the dermis
B are premalignant
C almost always regress spontaneously
D are most satisfactorily treated with superficial radiotherapy
E should be surgically excised

79 Fibroadenomata of the breast

A are commonest in early adult life
B are indiscrete and difficult to distinguish
C are usually painless
D are commonly associated with neurofibromata elsewhere
E resolve without treatment

77 A **True** Solar radiation is the most common cause.
   B **False** While this is so in squamous cell carcinomas, metastases are very rare in basal cell lesions.
   C **False** They are approximately three times more common.
   D **False** These are characteristic of squamous cell carcinomas. The classical appearance in basal cell lesions is of darkly staining solid masses of cells arising from the basal layer of epidermis.
   E **False** Such lesions are rare in oriental and almost unknown in black races. They typically occur in 'sun-worshipping' blonde subjects and on the exposed skin of outdoor workers.

78 A **True** They are raised, reddish-purple dermal vascular malformations.
   B **False** They have no malignant potential.
   C **True** The vast majority will spontaneously regress by 3 years of age. If this does not occur then a short dose of steroids may initiate regression.
   D **False** Radiotherapy for this or any other benign lesion is to be condemned because of the possible dangers of ensuing malignancies.
   E **False** Surgery is rarely necessary. Capillary angiomas should be distinguished from cavernous angiomas which develop from larger vessels. The latter appear in childhood, do not regress and frequently require surgical treatment.

79 A **True** The peak incidence is in the third decade.
   B **False** They are firm, smooth, well circumscribed, mobile lumps.
   C **True** In the majority of patients this is so.
   D **False** They are not neural structures and are usually solitary.
   E **True** Some tend to enlarge, but the majority resolve.

80   Fibrocystic disease of the breast
    A is a variant of the normal cyclical changes that the breast undergoes during menstruation
    B is normally unilateral
    C tends to progress in the postmenopausal years
    D is precancerous
    E is not usually painful

81   The management of fibrocystic breast disease should
    A usually be by surgical excision
    B include mammography when available
    C include therapy with oestrogens
    D include therapy with progesterone
    E requires, in the premenopausal patient, annual review

82   An intraduct papilloma of the breast
    A may cause a bloody nipple discharge
    B may be diagnosed with the aid of contrast radiography
    C should be treated by simple mastectomy
    D is associated with fibrocystic disease of the breast
    E is an indicator of an associated often occult carcinoma of the breast.

FIBROCYSTIC DISEASE

80 A **True**   There is glandular hyperplasia, cyst formation, duct
                   wall hyperplasia, periductal fibrosis and lymphocytic
                   infiltration.
    B **False** It is usually bilateral and most common in the upper
                   outer quadrant of the breasts.
    C **False** Though it is most common in the later years of
                   reproductive life, some regression and decrease in
                   pain occurs after the menopause.
    D **True**   There is an increase in the incidence of breast cancer
                   in those cases which reveal adenosis and metaplasia
                   of the breast epithelium.
    E **False** Pain is a frequent presenting symptom and is worse
                   premenstrually. — ? el Cold cycle

81 A **False** This is an extremely common condition and the
                   majority of patients are treated symptomatically.
                   Only when the lesion is discrete and carcinoma is
                   suspected is an excision biopsy undertaken.
    B **True**   Where this facility exists, advantage should be taken
                   of its ability to distinguish breast cancer from
                   fibrocystic disease. It may also detect a neoplasm
                   whose diagnosis is obscured by surrounding (and
                   unrelated) fibrocystic disease of the breast.
    C **False** These do not influence the progress of the disease
    D **False** although some pain relief may be achieved.
    E **False** Although the incidence of subsequent neoplasia is
                   increased, it is more practical to teach self-
                   examination and only review when changes occur.

INTRADUCTAL PAPILLOMA

82 A **True**   This and the occurrence of pain are the most
                   frequent symptoms.
    B **True**   Injection of the relevant duct with contrast medium
                   often confirms the diagnosis.
    C **False** Local removal of this benign lesion with or without
                   segmental resection of the breast is all that is
                   required.
    D **False** This benign neoplasm is not to be confused with the
                   diffuse papillomatous lesions often seen in
                   fibrocystic breast disease.
    E **False** No evidence exists linking it with breast cancer.

83 Paget's disease of the nipple
A usually presents as a bilateral eczema of the nipple
B is always related to an underlying breast cancer
C indicates incurable breast cancer
D has non-specific histological characteristics
E is a disease of younger women

84 The incidence of breast cancer
A increases with age
B decreases after premenopausal oophorectomy
C is relatively low in Japan
D is related to uterine cancer
E is related to dietary factors

85 Breast cancer
A is the commonest female neoplasm in the United Kingdom
B has its highest incidence in social class V
C has a familial tendency
D is less common in nulliparous women
E frequently presents as a breast cyst

83 A **False** It is usually a unilateral disease.
    B **True**   The lesion is an intraduct carcinoma arising in the
                  minute ducts of the nipple. It infiltrates the skin and
                  often extends deeply to produce a palpable mass.
    C **False** There is a good prognosis in these tumours
                  compared to other breast cancers. This is probably
                  related to earlier diagnosis and treatment.
    D **False** The histology is characteristic, viz: large clear
                  vacuolated cells (Paget's cells) invading the dermis,
                  epidermal hypertrophy and dermal lymphocytic
                  infiltration.
    E **False** Its incidence, like breast cancer, increases with age.

---

84 A **True**   There is an increasing incidence with age after
                  puberty.
    B **True**   Oophorectomy before 40 years of age considerably
                  reduced the expected incidence.
    C **True**   The incidence in Japan is less than 20 per cent of that
                  in Britain and the USA.
    D **False** No causal or associated relationship has been shown
                  to exist.
    E **True**   A diet high in animal fat is positively related to the
                  incidence of breast cancer.

---

85 A **True**   Followed by large bowel and uterine cancer.
    B **False** The highest incidence is in social class 1.
    C **True**   A maternal history or a history of a sibling with the
                  disease increases the incidence of breast cancer
                  compared with that of the general population.
    D **False** Nulliparous women have the highest incidence of
                  breast cancer, followed by those who did not have
                  their first child until 25 years of age. Breast feeding
                  seems to confer some slight protection.
    E **False** The majority are solid tumours. Rarely it may be
                  cystic and those that contain bloodstained fluid and
                  readily refill after aspiration merit suspicion and
                  biopsy.

86 Breast cancer

F **A** often presents with a history of breast pain
T **B** is most common in the upper outer quadrant of the breast
T **C** can be diagnosed preoperatively by the experienced clinician in 95 per cent of cases
T **D** must be considered on discovering any discrete mass in the breast
T **E** has an increased incidence in patients who have taken the contraceptive pill

87 The signs and symptoms of breast cancer include

F **A** a milky nipple discharge
T **B** eczematous changes in the nipple and areola
F **C** premenstrual breast pain
T **D** skin tethering
F **E** cyclical swelling of the breast

88 Radiological examination of the breast (mammography)

A does not improve the clinician's diagnosis rate of benign and malignant breast disease F
B is diagnostically most useful in young women   F
C is practical as a nationwide presymptomatic screening procedure in the United Kingdom T
D contributes nothing to the management of the patients with clinically obvious breast cancer F
E may be helpful in postoperative assessment of breast cancer patients T

86 A **True**   Though a painless lump is the first sign in two-thirds of patients, in more than 15 per cent pain is the presenting symptom.

   B **True**   Half the breast cancers occur in the upper outer quadrant and only 5 per cent in the lower inner quadrant. Medial lesions are much less common.

   C **False**   Most studies show clinical diagnosis to be accurate
   D **True**   in only 70 per cent of cases – thus all discrete non-cystic breast lumps must be subjected to biopsy.

   E **False**   This topic has been studied extensively. There is no evidence that the incidence is increased in these patients.

87 A **False**   Cancer should be suspected if a nipple discharge is bloodstained.

   B **True**   Paget's disease of the nipple, which produces eczematous changes in the nipple, is always associated with an underlying breast cancer.

   C **False**   This usually indicates fibrocystic disease of the breast. *PREMENSTRUAL PAIN*

   D **True**   This is best observed in the skin directly over the tumour. Apart from cancer only acute inflammation and fat necrosis show this sign.

   E **False**   In the premenstrual woman this is a normal phenomenon. Neoplasia does not produce this pre- or postmenstrually.

88 A **False**   The diagnosis rate is improved by 10 to 15 per cent.
   B **False**   The active young breast is relatively radio-opaque and the infiltrating opacification and punctate calcification of breast cancer are rendered more difficult to see.

   C **True**   It is probably best at present to confine it to women above the age of 50 years when cancer is more common and relatively easier to diagnose radiologically.

   D **False**   Mammography may reveal impalpable cancers and thus bilateral cancers will be diagnosed twice as frequently.

   E **True**   There is an increased incidence of second breast cancers in those patients who survive several years after treatment of their first. Mammography is recommended on the remaining breast every 3 years.

89 The histological study of breast cancers has shown that
   A   the prognosis is not related to histological type   F
   B   the commonest carcinoma is a squamous carcinoma   F
   C   most breast cancers arise from the epithelium of the breast
          lobule   T
   D   satellite breast cancers are common F
   E   the degree of differentiation is related to the prognosis

37/80

90 The prognosis of treated Stage I and Stage II breast cancer
   A   cannot be satisfactorily assessed until 15 years have elapsed
   B   is adversely affected by a subsequent pregnancy F
   C   is worse in the male
   D   is worse if the cancer is discovered during late pregnancy or
          the puerperium
   E   may be improved by tamoxifen

37/85

89 A **False**   Study of untreated patients with breast cancer
                    reveals that the prognosis is related to the
                    histological type. Medullary carcinoma, which is least
                    invasive, has the best prognosis.
    B **False**   The vast majority are adenocarcinomas.
    C **False**   Breast cancers arise from the nipple, the ducts or the
                    lobule epithelium. Duct cancer is by far the
                    commonest.
    D **True**   This is well marked in the commonest tumour – the
                    infiltrating adenocarcinoma (scirrhous carcinoma)
                    where early invasion of blood and lymph vessels
                    occurs.
    E **True**   Anaplastic tumours have the worst prognosis, well-
                    differentiated ones the best.

---

90 A **True**   The vast majority of recurrent breast neoplasms
                    occur in the first 15 years after treatment. Survival
                    rate after 15 years parallels that of a comparable age
                    group in the general population.
    B **False**   The survival rate is significantly improved in those
                    patients who become pregnant after treatment for
                    breast cancer (although oestrogens have a
                    deleterious effects in advanced breast neoplasia in
                    this age group).
    C **False**   Stage for stage, survival rates are similar in the two
                    sexes, but early spread to adjoining tissues renders
                    more male breast cancers surgically incurable.
    D **True**   The survival rate is about 5 per cent below that of
                    matched groups of non-pregnant patients.
    E **True**   The oestrogen antagonist tamoxifen will improve
                    survival if given for 2 years postoperatively to the
                    postmenopausal woman.

91   The prognosis of treated breast cancer is

A   related to the clinical staging of the cancer T

B   related to the number of axillary nodes found to be invaded by cancer at operation T

C   related to the use of postoperative radiotherapy to the regional nodes and operative field of the mastectomy

D   better after simple rather than radical mastectomy F

E   related to the histological appearance of the cancer T

92   In a patient with breast neoplasia distant metastases may be revealed by

A   a radiographic skeletal survey

B   a raised serum alkaline phosphatase

C   raised urinary 17-ketosteroid metabolites

D   a raised serum glutamic oxaloacetic transminase (SGOT)

E   a radioisotope bone scan

91 A **True**   When treated, approximately 65 per cent of patients
with Stage I (Manchester Classification) are alive
after 5 years, whereas survival rates of Stages II, III
and IV are progressively worse.

B **True**   When only two or three nodes are found to contain
tumour and these are removed, survival rates
approach those of Stage I. More than four affected
nodes worsens the prognosis considerably.

C **False**   No improvement in longevity following regional
radiotherapy as an adjuvant to mastectomy has been
found in patients with breast cancer. Local recurrence
of the disease is however diminished.

D **False**   Survival and recurrence rate appear to be similar in
the various methods of treatment of 'operable' breast
cancer. This similarity reflects the inadequacies of
clinical staging in that the consequences of occult,
unidentified metastases may disguise the small
differences between the various methods of
treatment.

E **True**   Poorly differentiated tumours have the worst
prognosis.

92 A **True**   Although almost half the patients presenting with
    B **True**   breast cancer have occult, and at present mostly
    C **False**   unidentifiable, metastatic deposits, a careful clinical
    D **True**   examination and some routine investigations will
    E **True**   reveal some of these deposits. A chest X-ray and a
skeletal survey will reveal some of the chest and
bone secondaries, and tho serum alkaline
phosphatase and SGOT may be elevated with liver
deposits. No serum or urinary factor at present
estimated is diagnostic of widespread disease. It is
debatable whether radioisotope scanning of the
bones and liver, athough they will reveal some
metastatic deposits, are justifiable as a routine
measure as yet because of their diagnostic
limitations.

93 Signs of incurable breast cancer include

A tumour fixity to the chest wall
B skin ulceration
C palpably enlarged mobile ipsilateral axillary lymph nodes
D a bloody nipple discharge
E diagnosis during pregnancy

94 Palliation of advanced incurable breast cancer

A can be achieved by therapy with anti-oestrogens
B can be achieved by oestrogen administration in the premenopausal patient
C can be achieved by androgen administration in the postmenopausal patient
D can be achieved by chemotherapeutic agents in pre- and postmenopausal patients
E may be achieved by radiotherapy

93 A **True**   These two signs together with peau d'orange,
    B **True**   lymphoedema of the arm and fixed axillary lymph
               nodes usually indicate incurable advanced cancer of
               the breast.
    C **False** More than half the enlarged axillary nodes associated
               with a breast neoplasm contain no tumour. This may
               be the result of an immune response to the tumour.
    D **False** A bloody discharge may indicate a benign papilloma,
               a ductal cancer, or invasion of a major duct by cancer
               but it need not indicate advanced or incurable
               disease.
    E **False** Though pregnancy often renders diagnosis difficult
               all studies show that the outcome and treatment is
               not worse at this time.

94 A **True**   This should be the first procedure to be tried –
               approximately one-third of patients will respond,
               especially those who are postmenopausal.
    B **False** In this group oestrogens often have a stimulatory
               effect on the cancer. Oestrogen-containing
               contraceptive pills are thus contraindicated.
    C **True**   About 20 per cent of patients will respond.
    D **True**   Single agents such as 5-fluorouracil and quadruple
               chemotherapy with added cyclophosphamide,
               vincristine and methotrexate have been shown to
               produce moderately high remission rates in both
               groups of patients.
    E **True**   Radiotherapy has a useful palliative role particularly
               when pain is caused by bone or soft tissue
               involvement, when there is superior vena cava
               obstruction or when the primary tumour is fungating.

6 Thyroid, parathyroid and adrenal glands

95 Signs and symptoms of hyperthyroidism include
A decreased sweating F
B an irregular pulse rate T
C cardiac failure T
D diplopia ? → ophthalmoplegia.   4/5
E pretibial myxoedema T

96 Symptoms of hyperthyroidism include
A intolerance to cold F
B increased appetite T   4/5
C emotional instability T
D diarrhoea T
E loss of visual acuity ?

97 Medical therapy of hyperthyroidism
A is particularly indicated in the pregnant patient ?
B will usually produce a long-lasting remission rate of 70 to 80 per cent after a 6-month course T
C is occasionally complicated by bone marrow depression T
D depends on the efficacy of the drugs in inhibiting the hypothalamic centres which govern thyroid stimulating hormone (TSH) release by the pituitary F
E may include the use of beta-adrenergic blocking agents T

1/x

9/15

95 A **False** There is increased sweating, producing the characteristic warm sweaty palms of the thyrotoxic patient.
    B **True**   Atrial fibrillation is particularly common in the elderly
    C **True**   and the deleterious effects on the cardiac output may produce cardiac failure in this group of patients.
    D **True**   Multiple eye signs of this condition include exophthalmos, lid lag and ophthalmoplegia, producing the characteristic facies of the severely thyrotoxic patient.
    E **True**   The skin below the knee is thickened and infiltrated with mucopolysaccharide giving non-pitting indurated plaques.

96 A **False** Amongst the host of symptoms, the most
    B **True**   characteristic is weight loss associated with an increased appetite.
    C **True**   There is marked heat intolerance and the development of irritability and emotional instability.
    D **True**   Diarrhoea and amenorrhoea may be prominent.
    E **True**   Visual acuity may deteriorate with papilloedema, retinal oedema and optic nerve damage.

97 A **False** These drugs may cross the placental barrier and inhibit fetal thyroid function. They may also be excreted in breast milk.
    B **False** Recurrence of hyperthyroidism after drug withdrawal occurs in up to 70 per cent of patients.
    C **True**   Both propylthiouracil and carbimazole produce agranulocytosis in a small number of patients. Drug rashes and hepatitis also occur.
    D **False** The thiouracil group of drugs acts by interfering with the organic binding of iodine; carbimazole by interfering with tri-iodothyronine synthesis in the gland.
    E **True**   Propanolol will control mild hyperthyroidism and is frequently used to prepare these patients for surgery.

98   Treatment of hyperthyroidism with radioactive iodine

T   **A**   is complicated by the late occurrence of thyroid cancer
F   **B**   should not be undertaken in patients below the age of 40
    C   is frequently complicated by the development of
           myxoedema
T   **D**   is often complicated by a short-lived exacerbation of the
           hyperthyroid state
T   **E**   is often followed by the need for maintenance treatment with
           thyroxine

− 2

7/20

99   The surgical treatment of hyperthyroidism

T   **A**   is commonly followed by hypothyroidism
F   **B**   has a high rate of recurrence
F   **C**   can be safely effected without preoperative drug therapy
T   **D**   may be complicated by postoperative high parathormone
           levels
T   **E**   may be complicated by subglottic oedema

8/25

98 A **False**   Cumulative experience and close study of patients in
    B **True**   the 30 years since the introduction of therapy with
                   radioactive iodine reveals no increased risk of
                   neoplasia. It is advisable however to restrict its use to
                   those patients in the latter half of life.
    C **True**   This may not develop for several years after
    D **True**   treatment and the incidence of hypothyroidism
                   seems to vary in different centres. Hypothyroidism
                   rates of 40 per cent 10 years after treatment are
                   common and this fraction increases with the passage
                   of time.
    E **False**   The treatment has no stimulant effect on the gland.
                   Its beneficial effects are not usually seen for a month
                   or two after ingestion of the radioactive iodine.

99 A **False**   Postoperative hypothyroidism can be detected in 5 to
    B **False**   10 per cent of patients. There is a similar incidence of
                   recurrent thyrotoxicosis.
    C **False**   To operate on the hyperthyroid gland is to court the
                   life-threatening condition of 'thyroid crisis' – acute
                   severe hyperthyroidism. The patient must be
                   rendered euthyroid preoperatively with antithyroid
                   drugs and/or beta-blockers such as propanolol.
    D **False**   Postoperative hypoparathyroidism occurs in a small
                   proportion of patients either due to disturbance to
                   the blood supply of the parathyroids or their
                   inadvertent removal.
    E **True**   This is frequently a consequence of postoperative
                   haemorrhage deep to the strap muscles.

100   A multinodular (adenomatous) goitre
- **A**   is more common in those patients having a deficient iodine intake
- **B**   is usually preceded by a diffuse goitre in early adult life
- **C**   may become neoplastic
- **D**   may be effectively treated with thyroid hormones
- **E**   rarely needs surgical treatment

101   Autoimmune thyroiditis (Hashimoto's disease)
- **A**   characteristically occurs in young females
- **B**   often presents with hyperthyroidism
- **C**   produces a soft diffuse enlargement of the thyroid gland
- **D**   is associated with regional lymph node enlargement
- **E**   is associated with raised serum levels of thyroid antibodies

102   Hashimoto's disease
- **A**   is often associated with increased levels of circulating thyroid antibodies
- **B**   is characterised by lymphocytic infiltration and fibrosis of the thyroid gland
- **C**   is usually treated by sub-total thyroidectomy
- **D**   should be treated by anti-thyroid drugs
- **E**   is frequently followed by thyroid cancer

100 A **True**   This has given rise to the term 'endemic goitre' for it refers to the high incidence of multinodular goitre in those areas low in naturally occurring iodine, e.g. Derbyshire in the United Kingdom, Switzerland and the Andes.

    B **True**   TSH stimulation, secondary to the iodine deficiency, results initially in diffuse hyperplasia. This is followed years later by the development of nodules of hyperplastic gland interposed with areas of involution and fibrosis

    C **True**   Approximately 5 per cent of multinodular goitres develop malignancies.

    D **True**   Thyroid hormone administration suppresses the effect of TSH on the adenomatous gland. In the early stages of the disease iodine can halt the development of a multinodular goitre from diffuse glandular enlargement.

    E **False**   Surgery is indicated when there is retrosternal extension, tracheal deviation, hyperthyroidism, or a dominant nodule which is suspicious of malignancy.

---

101 A **False**   It occurs most frequently in middle-aged females.

    B **True**   This is usually mild and short lived and is followed by the development of permanent hypothyroidism.

    C **False**   Diffuse enlargement of the gland does occur, but the gland is firm and rubbery.

    D **False**   Lymphadenopathy is not a feature of Hashimoto's disease and if present should arouse suspicion of thyroid neoplasia.

    E **True**   Thyroid antibodies are raised in autoimmune thyroid disease (e.g. Hashimoto's, thyroiditis and hyperthyroidism); raised levels may also be seen in malignancy.

---

102 A **True**   There is often a raised titre of anti-thyroglobulin antibodies and antibodies against thyroid acinar cells.

    B **True**   Fibrosis is a manifestation of the later stages of the disease.

    C **False**   The appropriate treatment is very individual. It is advisable to take an open thyroid biopsy; pressure on the trachea may demand excision of the thyroid isthmus and very occasionally cosmetic considerations require a sub-total thyroidectomy.

    D **False**   Thyroid hormones usually have to be given to combat hypothyroidism.

    E **False**   Thyroid cancers do not develop but there appears to be a very small chance that lymphomas of the thyroid may follow this diagnosis.

103 Thyroid cancer
  A frequently produces multinodular enlargement of the gland
  B should be diagnosed by preoperative needle biopsy of the gland
  C can be excluded if there is a localised but soft enlargement of the gland
  D often produces a bruit over the gland
  E may cause vocal cord palsy

104 Papillary carcinoma of the thyroid
  A may follow radiation exposure in childhood
  B is a slow-growing tumour
  C usually metastasises to lymph nodes
  D is usually a multifocal tumour
  E is rarely cured by surgery

105 Follicular carcinoma of the thyroid
  A is most common in females
  B is most common above the age of 30 years
  C usually metastasises to lymph nodes
  D is associated with a relatively good prognosis in childhood
  E is best treated by near total thyroidectomy

103 A **False** Whilst cancer occasionally develops in a multinodular goitre the usual signs of thyroid neoplasia are a localised or generalised swelling of the gland.

B **False** Although it is difficult to diagnose well-differentiated cancers from a small biopsy specimen, poorly differentiated lesions can be diagnosed by skilled cytologists.

C **False** Well-differentiated lesions frequently present as soft solitary swellings. All solitary swellings of the gland should have an excision biopsy performed.

D **False** There is no hypervascularity in thyroid cancer.

E **True** In the absence of previous thyroid surgery recurrent nerve palsy almost always indicates a malignant goitre.

104 A **True** This is most marked in cancers appearing before adolescence. A history of irradiation has been noted in 70 per cent of papillary cancers in this age group.

B **True** This is particularly so in young patients where growth of the primary and metastases is slow.

C **True** Whilst this is the most common mode of spread, spread by the bloodstream is not uncommon in the older patient.

D **True** This is frequently noted and may represent intraglandular spread.

E **False** Intrathyroid tumours have a 10-year survival rate of 90 per cent after resection and 50 per cent of those that spread to lymph nodes are cured by resection.

105 A **True** As is papillary carcinoma.

B **True** Whereas papillary carcinoma is most common in children and younger adults.

C **False** Although lymphatic spread does occur, spread by the bloodstream to bones and lungs is more frequent.

D **True** There is an increased incidence of well-differentiated, well-encapsulated follicular and papillary carcinomas in this age group and they are associated with a good prognosis.

E **True** This approach has advantages over lobectomy; it ensures the removal of multifocal cancers and permits postoperative radiation scanning in the search for secondaries.

106   Undifferentiated carcinoma of the thyroid
  A   is most common in females
  B   is most common above the age of 60 years
  C   is often thyroid stimulating hormone (TSH) dependent
  D   often exhibits independent thyroid hormone production
  E   is always preceded by a long-standing goitre

107   The surgical treatment of thyroid cancer
  A   should be by 'near total' thyroidectomy in the potentially curable patient
  B   should include a frozen section histological examination of the tumour
  C   should include block dissection of the neighbouring lymph nodes whether or not they appear to contain tumour
  D   is most successful in the papillary type of cancer
  E   should be preceded by a therapeutic dose of I^{131}

108   Recurrent thyroid cancer can effectively be treated by
  A   high doses of I^{131}
  B   high doses of thyroid hormone
  C   extenal irradiation
  D   chemotherapy
  E   further surgery

106   A   **False**   There is an equal incidence in the two sexes.
      B   **True**   It rarely occurs before this age.
      C   **False**   The histological picture is of sheets of undifferentiated
      D   **False**   cells with no follicular formation. No evidene of
                      hormonal activity or response to hormonal therapy
                      exists in this type of tumour.
      E   **True**   In all cases the patient gives a history of a goitre with
                      a rapid, recent growth of a nodule within it.

107   A   **True**   Many of the tumours are multifocal and only the
                      posterior rim of thyroid tissue (and associated
                      parathyroid glands) on the opposite side of the neck
                      to the primary tumour should be preserved.
      B   **True**   A papillary tumour will be readily recognised and the
                      thyroidectomy must include clearance of the pre- and
                      paratracheal nodes, since they are frequently
                      involved. Follicular tumours, of which not so many
                      will be diagnosed at surgery, are initially treated by
                      total lobectomy alone. Near total removal of the
                      gland also allows a postoperative search for active
                      metastases by an I^{131} scan.
      C   **False**   Removal of the near total gland, allows postoperative
                      search for active metastases by an I^{131} scan.
      D   **True**   The histological type and the presence or absence of
                      invasion are of great significance in determining the
                      outcome after surgical treatment. Long term survival
                      has been frequently recorded in incompletely
                      removed papillary and follicular carcinomata of the
                      thyroid where these are well differentiated, whereas
                      undifferentiated cancers are uniformly fatal whatever
                      the treatment.
      E   **False**   Histological diagnosis may be interfered with. I^{131} has
                      no part to play in preoperative therapy.

108   A   **True**   A therapeutic dose of radioactive iodine is the
      B   **True**   treatment of choice. TSH suppression by means of
                      thyroid hormones is used in well-differentiated
                      tumours with good results.
      C   **True**   External irradiation is of value in palliating
                      undifferentiated tumours and lymphomas.
      D   **False**   There are as yet no reports of satisfactory remission
                      rates being produced by chemotherapy.
      E   **True**   The lymph node recurrences of papillary cancers can
                      be simply and effectively treated by local excision.

109   The earliest symptoms of hyperparathyroidism include

A   diarrhoea
B   polydipsia and polyuria
C   unexplained weight gain
D   muscle spasm
E   bone pains

110   Primary hyperparathyroidism

A   is most common in postmenopausal females
B   is occasionally diagnosed by routine biochemical screening
     of patients
C   should be considered when a patient presents with tetany
D   can be caused by adenomas or hyperplasia of the glands
E   may be diagnosed by radiographs of the hand

**111   Skeletal signs, symptoms and radiological evidence of
       hyperparathyroidism**

A   include demineralisation of the bones
B   include bone cysts and osteoclastoma formation
C   include spontaneous fractures
D   are the most common presenting complaints
E   include delayed union of fractures

109 A **False** The earliest symptoms are vague and rarely suggest
    B **True**   the diagnosis but constipation, muscle weakness,
    C **False** bone pains, anorexia and weight loss together with
    D **False** thirst and polyuria are encountered.
    E **True**

110 A **True**   It is three times more common in females and
particularly frequent between 45 and 65 years of age.
It is rare in children.

    B **True**   The rate of recognition has increased since
biochemical screening has been introduced. A raised
serum calcium, particularly if associated with a low
serum phosphate, is a strong pointer to the
diagnosis.

    C **False** Tetany only occurs with a low serum calcium. The
commonest presenting symptoms are vague
abdominal and bone pains. Fractures are not
uncommon and renal calculi may produce renal or
ureteric colic. Thus the adage; hyperparathyroidism
equals 'groans, bones and stones'.

    D **True**   Since adenomata are the most common cause of the
condition. Generalised hyperplasia may cause
hyperparathyroidism. Carcinoma is very rarely
encountered.

    E **True**   Subperiosteal bone resorption in the middle and
terminal phalanges is diagnostic of the condition.

111 A **True**   This is a general phenomenon affecting the whole
skeleton.

    B **True**   This is particularly common in the bones of the lower
limbs and ribs.

    C **True**   These indicate advanced and severe
hyperparathyroidism.

    D **False** The most common presenting signs and symptoms
are those referrable to the renal tract.

    E **False** Though the weakened bones fracture easily their
healing is unimpaired.

112 Renal symptoms of hyperparathyroidism

A   may be due to renal stones
B   may be due to nephrocalcinosis
C   are frequently those of chronic renal failure
D   are associated with hypertension
E   are associated with a high serum phosphate

113 Acute adrenal insufficiency

A   in the newborn is due to haemorrhage into one or both adrenal glands
B   in the newborn typically occurs in the second week of life
C   in the adult usually follows a pneumococcal septicaemia
D   in the adult is most frequently encountered following bilateral adrenalectomy
E   may occur after childbirth

114 Phaeochromocytomas

A   are tumours of the spinal nerve roots
B   are frequently multiple
C   characteristically present with a lemon-yellow skin discolouration
D   produce excessive amounts of catecholamines
E   can be effectively managed by long term medical therapy

112 A **True** Renal stones occur in over half the patients.
B **True** Nephrocalcinosis is less common, about 5 per cent of patients being affected.
C **True** More than 70 per cent of patients have renal damage and this may be severe especially when nephrocalcinosis is present.
D **True** More than 70 per cent of patients have hypertension and in the majority this is associated with renal damage.
E **False** Phosphate levels are low in hyperparathyroidism.

113 A **True** Adrenal apoplexy in the newborn is usually fatal
B **False** within the first few days of life. Haemorrhage into the glands occurs at birth and is possibly precipitated by withdrawal of maternal hormones. The condition is sometimes associated with birth trauma.
C **False** While streptococcal, staphylococcal and pneumococcal septicaemia may all give rise to the Waterhouse–Friderichsen syndrome it is most commonly associated with fulminating meningococcal septicaemia.
D **False** This should be prevented by the routine administration of steroid replacement during and after the operation.
E **True** Pituitary infarction occasionally occurs then and almost always subsequently results in acute adrenal insufficiency.

114 A **False** They arise from chromaffin cells of the adrenal medulla and the sympathetic nervous system.
B **True** 40 per cent are multiple.
C **False** The characteristic symptoms are due to intermittent catecholamine release and thus all the symptoms and signs of sympathetic overactivity such as paroxysmal tachycardia, flushing, sweating and palpitations are intermittently produced. Hypertension will eventually become permanent and diabetes is often present.
D **True** These, and their major breakdown product vanillyl mandelic acid (VMA) can be measured in a 24-hour urine specimen. CT scanning is useful to localise the tumour preoperatively.
E **False** Prompt surgical treatment is the rule. During the operation undue handling of the tumour may result in a very serious tachycardia and a dangerous attack of hypertension. These problems are reduced by effective preoperative sympathetic blockade.

115 Cushing's syndrome
- **A** is usually accompanied by an increased deposition of fat over the face and trunk
- **B** is most frequently due to an adrenal tumour
- **C** may be associated with bronchogenic cancer
- **D** is effectively treated with total bilateral adrenalectomy, even when shown to be pituitary dependent
- **E** should be managed medically unless complications develop

116 A thyroglossal cyst
- **A** usually presents in middle age
- **B** is a remnant of fifth pharyngeal arch mesoderm
- **C** should usually be excised with the thyroid cartilage
- **D** does not move with swallowing
- **E** may present as a neck abscess

115 A **True**   Facial and truncal adiposity, polycythaemia, diabetes and skin striae are characteristic findings. The serum potassium is invariably high and hypertension is common.

  B **False**   More than half the cases studied show the causitive lesion to be in the pituitary. This liberates ACTH and stimulates the adrenals into overactivity.

  C **True**   Ectopic ACTH may be produced by several neoplasms of which the lung is the commonest.

  D **True**   This is usually successful. There is a high rate of recurrence if a subtotal adrenalectomy is performed.

  E **False**   There is, as yet, no curative medical treatment and, since the patient progressively worsens, surgical treatment is always advised.

116 A **False**   They most frequently appear before adulthood and one-third of them appear before the age of 10 years.

  B **False**   The thyroid develops as a downgrowth from the back of the tongue into the third and fourth pharyngeal arches. A thyroglossal cyst is a remnant along the course of this tract.

  C **False**   But it is usually necessary to remove the body of the hyoid bone in order to follow, and remove, the tract into the base of the tongue.

  D **False**   Like the thyroid gland it moves with the larynx in swallowing.

  E **True**   They are prone to infection. Simple incision of the abscess is usually followed by a discharging sinus.

7 Oral cavity, pharynx and oesophagus

117 Surgical repair of a cleft lip and palate
    A should not be undertaken until the child begins to talk
    B is essential for normal feeding of the child
    C is essential to ensure normal development of speech
    D should frequently be combined with dental prosthetic work
    E may be associated with hearing disorders

118 Salivary duct calculi
    A produce pain on eating
    B are commonest in the parotid ducts
    C are a common cause of acute parotitis
    D are associated with hypercalcaemic states
    E often require excision of the affected salivary gland

117   A   **False**   Early closure of the defects is desirable whatever
      B   **True**   their form; cleft lips at about 3 months and palates at
      C   **True**   9 to 12 months. In this way suckling difficulties are
                      overcome, there is a likelihood of normal voice
                      development and cosmetic deformities are
                      minimised.
      D   **True**   Bilateral palatal clefts often require staged surgical
                      correction and an occlusive dental palatal plate may
                      allow normal voice development.
      E   **True**   Disruption of the palatal musculature leads to
                      eustachian tube destruction and fluid retention in the
                      middle ear.

118   A   **True**   The increased production of salivary juice produces
                      painful distension of the gland.
      B   **False**   The submandibular salivary duct is far more
                      commonly affected.
      C   **False**   The common causes of acute parotitis are debility,
                      dehydration and poor oral hygiene.
      D   **False**   There is no evidence that generalised metabolic
                      disorders play any part in the formation of salivary
                      duct calculi. Their aetiology is obscure but may be
                      related to a disturbance in the pH of the saliva.
      E   **True**   Infection, commonest in the submandibular gland,
                      frequently demands gland excision when the stone is
                      trapped deep in the duct.

119   Salivary tumours
  A   are most commonly seen in the paroid gland
  B   of the parotid gland, producing facial nerve lesions, are
       usually malignant
  C   may appear as palatal swellings
  D   are in most cases satisfactorily treated by radiotherapy
  E   are usually benign

120   Cancer of the tongue
  A   is usually an adenocarcinoma
  B   is more common in males
  C   most commonly presents as an indolent ulcer
  D   metastasises via the lymphatics at an early stage of the
       disease
  E   is best treated by surgery and radiotherapy

119 A **True**   75 per cent of all salivary gland tumours occur in the parotid.

    B **True**   The majority of parotid tumours are benign (and of these, the commonest is the mixed parotid tumour – pleomorphic adenoma) but malignancy is likely if there is an associated facial nerve palsy, an infiltration of the overlying skin or cervical lymph node enlargement.

    C **True**   The small and numerous salivary glands of the palate may become neoplastic – the commonest tumour here being the highly malignant cylindroma.

    D **False**   Surgical excision is the basis of treatment. Radiotherapy is only required for the rare malignant lesions that recur or have been incompletely removed.

    E **True**   Although the commonest tumour, the pleomorphic adenoma, frequently recurs because surgical excision is often incomplete due to microscopic tongues of tumour that extend into the surrounding normal tissue.

120 A **False**   Although adenocarcinomas do occur, more than 95 per cent of tongue cancers are of squamous origin.

    B **True**   It occurs four times as frequently in males. There is often a history of chronic irritation, leukoplakia, chronic alcoholism or long-standing iron deficiency anaemia.

    C **True**   Infiltrative forms of the cancer are recognised but the commonest presentation is of a chronic painless ulcer.

    D **True**   More than half the patients have lymph node

    E **True**   deposits at the time of presentation and, with cancers of the dorsum of the tongue, these may be bilateral. Surgical excision of the primary tumour and affected lymph nodes forms the basis of treatment. This is usually supplemented with radiotherapy.

121 Pharyngeal pouches

A usually occur at the pharyngo-oesophageal junction
B are commonest in young people
C may cause pulmonary problems
D usually present with dysphagia
E usually require surgical excision

122 Pharyngo-oesophageal diverticula

A only occur at the level of cricopharyngeus
B may be related to para-oesophageal lymph nodes
C are often associated with recurrent attacks of pneumonitis
D characteristically present with vomiting
E can be associated with oesophageal motility problems

123 The diagnosis of oesophageal achalasia may be made by

A a carefully taken history of the patient's complaints
B oesophageal biopsy
C barium swallow X-ray examination
D oesophagoscopy
E oesophageal motility studies

121 A **False** The commonest site is to the left of the midline
              posteriorly, between the oblique fibres and the
              transverse cricopharyngeal portion of the inferior
              constrictor muscle of the pharynx.
     B **False** The majority occur in elderly patients.
     C **True**   Aspiration of the diverticular contents may occur,
              particularly at night, producing aspiration
              pneumonitis. In addition, dysphagia and gurgling
              during deglutition may be present.
     D **True**   The dysphagia is the presenting symptom in three-
              quarters of patients. Motor abnormalities in the
              upper oesophageal sphincter may play a part.
     E **True**   Excision of the diverticulum and closure of the
              pharyngeal wall is the usual method of treatment.

122 A **False** There are three common sites of occurrence, at the
     B **True**   level of cricopharyngeus, just above the diaphragm,
              and in the mid-oesophageal region.
     C **True**   Aspiration of oesophageal contents is a consequence
              of the larger diverticula. This occurs particularly at
              night.
     D **False** Regurgitation, noisy eating and dysphagia are the
              commonest symptoms.
     E **True**   Unco-ordinated oesophageal contractions are
              common in the elderly and not infrequently
              associated with epiphrenic diverticulae.

123 A **False** The patient complains of dysphagia but symptoms
              may be present for a few weeks or several years. The
              dysphagia of achalasia cannot be distinguished with
              certainty from that due to other conditions.
     B **False** The neurological changes lie submucosally and a
              deep biopsy would be needed. This is a dangerous
              procedure.
     C **True**   The characteristic finding is of a dilated oesophagus
              narrowing down in a conical fashion to a smooth
              stenosis of the cardia.
     D **True**   This will distinguish early achalasia from a benign
              stricture or cancer.
     E **True**   In advanced cases there is no peristalsis and no
              swallowing reflex present. The oesophagus empties
              purely by gravity.

124 In oesophageal achalasia
  A dysphagia is usually the first symptom
  B pain is rarely a prominent symptom
  C there is an absence of peristalsis in the oesophagus
  D there is an absence of ganglion cells in Auerbach's plexus in the wall of the oesophagus
  E the fundamental problem is spasm of cricopharyngeus F muscle

125 The treatment of oesophageal achalasia
  A is commonly by a cardiomyotomy (Heller's operation)
  B can be by dilation
  C should be by oesophagogastrectomy
  D should include a transthoracic vagotomy
  E may be successfully achieved by amyl nitrate or nifedipine

126 'Sideropaenic dysphagia'
  A is associated with koilonychia and atrophic oral mucosa
  B is a disease of elderly women
  C is related to long-standing Vitamin B_{12} deficiency
  D is also known eponymously as the 'Paterson–Kelly syndrome' or the 'Plummer–Vinson syndrome'
  E is usually due to an oesophageal cancer

124 A **True** This is often more marked for liquids than solids, and is eased by 'trick' swallowing manoeuvres by the patient.

B **False** In more than 25 per cent of cases the patient complains of diffuse retrosternal pain in the early stages of the disease. This decreases as the functional obstruction worsens.

C **True** The oesophagus is immobile, dilated and empties only by gravity through a lower oesophageal sphincter which does not relax (cardiospasm).

D **True** Whether this is a primary or secondary phenomenon is not known, but it is present in the majority of cases.

E **False** The motor abnormality is a failure of relaxation of the gastro-oesophageal sphincter.

125 A **True** Patients are helped by this procedure although postoperative reflux oesophagitis may occasionally be a problem.

B **True** The development of balloons with a preformed contour has markedly increased the use of this technique, surgery being reserved for failure and recurrences. Oesophageal perforation is an occasional complication of the procedure.

C **False** This is too extensive a procedure and is not rational since the stomach is free of any pathology.

D **False** Section of the vagus has no effect on oesophageal motility.

E **False** Though these drugs relax the lower oesophageal sphincter, they are not completely effective and have side-effects.

126 A **True** The majority of cases occur in middle-aged or elderly
B **True** women.
C **False** The majority of cases are associated with long-standing iron deficiency anaemia. The reason for this association is obscure.

D **True** It was first described in 1919 by Paterson and Kelly.
E **False** The commonest cause is a fibrous web occurring in the upper oesophagus. However, about 10 per cent of patients develop cancers of the oesophagus, pharynx or oral cavity.

127 The symptoms of peptic oesophagitis
A   include intermittent dysphagia
B   are often associated with those of anaemia
C   include retrosternal discomfort
D   are more likely to occur when the patient is in the upright position
E   can occur in childhood

128 Peptic oesophagitis
A   is effectively demonstrated by a barium swallow and meal
B   is always associated with a hiatus hernia
C   can be readily confirmed by oesophagoscopy
D   is associated with the production of higher than normal amounts of gastric acid
E   is a condition confined to adults

127 A **True**   Severe oesophagitis produces mucosal oedema and
                     spasm of the underlying oesophageal muscle. This is
                     often intermittent. Submucosal inflammatory
                     changes may eventually produce fibrosis and a
                     stricture of the lower end of the oesophagus. This is
                     often associated with an alleviation of the symptoms
                     of oesophagitis since reflux occurs less readily
                     through the stricture.
     B **True**   Chronic blood loss may occur from the inflamed and
                     haemorrhagic oesophageal mucosa.
     C **True**   Retrosternal discomfort is the commonest sympton
                     but discomfort also may be produced in the neck,
                     chest and epigastrium.
     D **False**   This position often relieves the discomfort, which is
                     usually produced by stooping and lying down.
     E **True**   A congenital sliding hiatus hernia often results in
                     severe reflux with oesophageal ulceration and
                     stricture.

128 A **False**   Though radiologists are often successful at
                     demonstrating a sliding hiatus hernia, it is known
                     that only some of these patients will have
                     oesophagitis.
     B **False**   Oesophagitis may also occur without a hernia being
                     demonstrated. The radiological demonstration of
                     oesophagitis is not usually possible unless spasm or
                     stenosis exists.
     C **True**   This is the most important investigation. The
                     inflamed mucosa can be recognised by its friability
                     and by contact bleeding. Occasionally ulceration of
                     the mucosa will be seen.
     D **False**   No relationship between acid output and
                     oesophagitis has been demonstrated. It may be that
                     bile salts are the noxious constituents of the fluid
                     reflux. There is no association with duodenal
                     ulceration.
     E **False**   Infants born with a congenital hiatus hernia suffer
                     from reflux and oesophagitis.

129   The successful medical management of peptic oesophagitis
  A   should include anticholinergic drugs
  B   includes weight reduction
  C   includes elevating the head of the bed
  D   depends on regular antacid administration
  E   may follow pharmacological reduction of gastric acidity

130   Surgical management of peptic oesophagitis
  A   is indicated in the majority of patients
  B   is based on the prevention of reflux
  C   is best restricted to repeated bouginage when peptic
       strictures are present
  D   should include a vagotomy
  E   may result in splenic damage

131   Para-oesophageal hiatus herniae
  A   usually occur through a defect in the diaphragm to the right
       of the oesophagus.
  B   usually have an easily recognised hernial sac
  C   usually have colon herniating alongside the oesophagus
  D   are usually accompanied by oesophagitis
  E   may produce postprandial chest pain

129 A **False** These are not helpful.
     B **True**   Weight reduction may reduce intra-abdominal
     C **True**   pressure but it only alleviates the symptoms slightly.
                   Elevation of the head of the bed is worthwhile,
                   especially in patients with mild symptoms. Regular
                   small meals and reduction in smoking are also of
                   benefit.
     D **True**   They provide symptomatic relief and may reduce
                   reflux by increasing the tone of the gastro-
                   oesophageal sphincter.
     E **True** H_2 blockade, and omeprazole have both been shown
                   to be effective in a large proportion of cases.

130 A **False** The necessary surgical procedure involves a major
                   abdominal or thoracic operation. It has a significant
                   morbidity and a small mortality. Only serious
                   symptoms are an indication for surgery.
     B **True**   Several surgical procedures exist and their rationale
                   is, in all cases, the prevention of reflux.
     C **False** Bouginage will provide only short term relief. It
                   permits reflux to recur with the recurrence of
                   oesophagitis. Bouginage combined with surgical
                   prevention of reflux is, however, very satisfactory
                   management.
     D **False** Adding vagotomy to an antireflux procedure does
                   not improve the results.
     E **True**   This is one of the common complications, splenic
                   tears follow traction in the upper abdomen.

131 A **False** The hernial ring is always on the left side of the
                   oesophagus.
     B **True**   These are true herniae of the fundus of the stomach
                   into the chest. The cardia remains in its usual
                   abdominal position.
     C **False** The colon is not involved in para-oesophageal
                   herniae.
     D **False** There is not usually any incompetence of the cardia
                   so reflux of gastric contents and oesophagitis do not
                   occur.
     E **True**   The distension of the intrathoracic portion of the
                   stomach after meals produces a severe 'crushing'
                   pain in the chest and this is often confused with
                   angina.

132 Para-oesophageal hiatus herniae

A   may produce angina-like symptoms
B   are frequently associated with gastric ulceration
C   are frequently accompanied by occult gastrointestinal blood
     loss
D   are congenital in origin
E   should be managed conservatively in the majority of patients

133 Cancer of the oesophagus

A   usually presents with intermittent dysphagia
B   has its highest incidence in the fifth decade
C   is reliably diagnosed by barium swallow
D   should be assessed endoscopically when surgical resection
     is contemplated
E   may require bronchoscopic assessment

134 Malignant tumours of the oesophagus

A   are most commonly adenocarcinomas
B   occur most commonly in males
C   are most commonly situated in its upper third
D   commonly spread by lymphatics
E   can be effectively treated with radiotherapy

132 A **True**   The compressing retrosternal pain after food is
               frequently mistaken for angina.
     B **True**   Ulceration of the portion of the stomach inside the
               hernia is common.
     C **True**   Bleeding occurs from gastric ulceration or the area of
               gastritis which is frequently present in the part of the
               stomach adjacent to the hernial ring.
     D **False** They are rarely seen before middle age and are most
               common in the elderly. It is generally assumed they
               are acquired lesions.
     E **False** Treatment is usually surgical and is often indicated
               because of the distressing symptoms, the chronic
               blood loss and the risk of strangulation or
               perforation.

133 A **False** The commonest symptom is a progressive
               unremitting dysphagia.
     B **False** The incidence rises with age and is most common in
               patients over 70.
     C **True**   Positive information is yielded by this investigation in
               more than 95 per cent of patients.
     D **True**   This allows biopsy or cytological examination of the
               lesion by oesophagoscopy.
     E **True**   Bronchoscopy should be performed to establish
               whether the trachea or bronchi are invaded by a
               tumour of the middle third of the oesophagus.

134 A **False** The squamous cell carcinoma is by far the
               commonest tumour. Adenocarcinomas are almost
               entirely confined to the lower end of the oesophagus
               where they arise from the columnar epithelium
               adjacent to the cardia.
     B **True**   Overall, these malignancies are between two and five
               times more frequent in males, although cancers of
               the upper third of the oesophagus occur
               predominantly in females.
     C **False** About half the malignancies occur in the middle third
               and about one-third in the lower third.
     D **True**   Intramural extension, spread to lymph nodes and
               local spread to invade adjacent structures are all very
               common. Blood-borne metastases are rare.
     E **True**   This is used palliatively but there is some evidence
               that radiotherapy could be of value as an adjuvant to
               surgery.

135 Vomiting against a closed glottis may
   A cause a 'spontaneous' rupture of the oesophagus
   B be followed by severe chest pain and circulatory collapse
   C be effectively managed conservatively
   D cause a laceration of the mucosa of the oesophagogastric junction
   E cause gastrointestinal bleeding

135 A **True**   There is a rapid increase in intraluminal pressure
    B **True**   which may be followed by rupture of the lower end
    C **False** of the oesophagus with expulsion of air and gastric
                contents into the mediastinum and pleural cavity
                (usually the left side). This condition is known as the
                Boerhaave syndrome after the name of the first
                recorded patient. Immediate surgical repair is
                required. The mortality is high.
    D **True**   This is known as the 'Mallory–Weiss' syndrome.
    E **True**   There is no pain associated with the bleeding;
                barium studies are not as helpful as endoscopy in
                diagnosis. Surgical measures are occasionally
                required to stop continuing bleeding.

8 Hernia, peritoneum and abdominal trauma

136 The diagnosis of an inguinal hernia

A in an infant often depends on the history given by its mother
B in the adult is most easily made with the patient in the sitting position
C depends on the hernial sac or cough impulse being felt below the inguinal ligament
D is supported by the presence of a transilluminable scrotal swelling
E is more frequently made in females than in males

137 Inguinal herniae in children

A are usually of the indirect type
B are congenital in origin
C will regress spontaneously
D frequently obstruct
E may be associated with a hydrocele

138 Strangulation of a hernial sac

A is always accompanied by intestinal obstruction
B is more common in direct than indirect inguinal herniae
C is usually irreducible
D produces local pain and tenderness
E demands surgical relief

136 A **True** An inguinal lump may have been noted only when the child is crying, therefore an isolated examination may not reveal it. A slight thickening of the spermatic cord caused by the empty hernial sac may be palpable.

B **False** The patient should have his groin inspected and palpated when standing.

C **False** Inguinal herniae are seen and felt to emerge through the superficial inguinal ring above the inguinal ligament, femoral herniae are found below it.

D **False** A hernia is not usually transilluminable (whereas epididymal cysts and hydroceles usually are).

E **False** Males outnumber females by more than 10 to 1.

137 A **True** The vast majority of inguinal herniae in childhood are
B **True** indirect inguinal herniae within a patient processus vaginalis.

C **False** They do not obliterate spontaneously and should be treated surgically.

D **True** Obstruction will occur in 20 per cent of patients before their first birthday.

E **True** A persistent hydrocele indicates a patent processus vaginalis which may contain a hernia.

138 A **False** Herniae may produce strangulation of omentum without intestinal involvement. Occasionally only part of the intestinal wall is 'threatened' (a Richter's hernia) and intestinal obstruction may not occur.

B **False** Direct inguinal herniae are less likely to strangulate for they have a wider neck and a shorter sac.

C **True** Irreducibility is a sign of incarceration of the hernial contents and strangulation may be imminent.

D **True** Strangulation produces pain, local tenderness and, often, discolouration of the overlying tissues.

E **True** Surgical relief is essential to avoid toxaemia, peritonitis and death.

139 Incisional herniae are related to
   A wound infections
   B anaemia and malnutrition
   C obesity
   D the use of absorbable suture materials
   E failure of surgical technique

140 Herniae in the umbilical region
   A are always acquired in origin
   B usually occur in males
   C usually require surgical repair in infants
   D rarely strangulate
   E should be treated by a surgical corset

139 A **True**   These are iatrogenic herniae and the commonest
     B **False** predisposing cause is an infection of the original
                   surgical wound.
     C **True**   There is a greatly increased incidence in obese
                   patients, possibly because of the increased incidence
                   of wound haematomata but no definite evidence
                   exists that either anaemia or hypoproteinaemia
                   contributes to their formation.
     D **True**   The use of absorbable suture materials to
                   approximate aponeurotic sheaths is, possibly, a
                   factor in their formation. Catgut loses its tensile
                   strength in 10 to 20 days and aponeuroses do not
                   gain more than 60 per cent of their original strength
                   for 6 to 8 months.
     E **True**   Underlying all the above causes may be poor
                   surgical technique (broken sutures, slipped knots,
                   sutures cutting out because of inadequate bite).

140 A **False** They are of two types: the infantile type which
                   presents at birth is due to a congenital weakness in
                   the umbilicus, and the acquired adult type which
                   most frequently occurs in obese elderly patients is
                   due to a weakness occurring in the linea alba just
                   above the umbilicus. This latter type is known as a
                   para-umbilical hernia.
     B **False** There is not an increased incidence in males.
     C **False** Those of the infantile type frequently close
                   spontaneously before the age of 2 years, especially if
                   the defect is less than 1 cm in diameter.
     D **False** The para-umbilical hernia is particularly prone to
                   strangulation, and surgical repair is thus usually
                   indicated in this group.
     E **False** Surgical repair should be recommended for all.
                   Trusses do not work.

141   A discharge from the umbilicus
A   may indicate a patent vitello-intestinal duct
B   may indicate an anomaly of the urachus
C   at the time of menstruation may indicate endometriosis
D   in the neonate is of no immediate clinical significance
E   appearing for the first time in the adult usually indicates poor personal hygiene

142   An exomphalos
A   is a congenital defect of the urethra
B   is a congenital defect of the anterior abdominal wall
C   results from a patent vitello-intestinal duct
D   is otherwise known as gastroschisis
E   needs urgent surgical treatment if the sac has ruptured

143   Widespread carcinomatous involvement of the peritoneum
A   is frequently confirmed by abdominal paracentesis
B   can often be diagnosed by rectal examination
C   indicates that the primary neoplasm is abdominal in origin
D   is usually associated with jaundice
E   is usually associated with constant abdominal pain

141 A **True**   When the vitello-intestinal duct fails to disappear and remains patent throughout its length, a congenital small bowel fistula exists. Other related anomalies include Meckel's diverticulum and a fibrous congenital vitello-intestinal band.

     B **True**   A patent urachus results in the intermittent discharge of urine from the umbilicus.

     C **True**   This is rare; the discharge is bloody and arises from ectopic endometrial tissue.

     D **False**   In addition to the congenital defects already referred to, infection of the umbilicus (omphalitis) in the new born is potentially dangerous because of its rapid spread to the surrounding abdominal wall, peritoneum and, via incompletely obliterated umbilical vessels, to the liver.

     E **True**   Adult omphalitis is usually caused by retained foreign material in the umbilical scar.

142 A **False**   Exomphalos is a herniation of intra-adominal viscera
     B **True**   through the umbilical ring. It is covered by a
     C **False**   peritoneal sac which often ruptures after birth.
     D **False**   Gastroschisis is a congenital defect of the abdominal wall and has no membranous covering. A proportion of the less severe cases can be treated by primary closure but the majority with an intact sac are treated by dressing with 2 per cent mercurochrome. This allows epithelialisation to occur and the ventral hernia can be treated at a later date.

     E **True**   A ruptured exomphalos or gastroschisis needs urgent closure. In the larger defects this may be achieved by covering with silastic sheeting which allows epithelialisation and staged closure to be undertaken.

143 A **True**   Cytological examination of a sample of ascitic fluid often reveals the presence of exfoliated neoplastic cells.

     B **True**   The rectovesical or recto-uterine pouch is frequently the site of peritoneal metastitic deposits.

     C **False**   Disseminated breast cancer frequently results in peritoneal deposits and ascites.

     D **False**   Although metastases in the liver and porta hepatis are frequently present, there is no close association between peritoneal deposits and jaundice.

     E **False**   Painless distension of the abdomen due to ascites is a frequent presentation.

144   Blunt injuries to the abdomen
A   may cause peritonitis
B   may cause intestinal obstruction
C   may cause acute gastroduodenal ulceration
D   rarely need urgent laparotomy
E   rarely cause damage to retroperitoneal structures

145   Car seat belts (lap diagonal) when properly adjusted
A   prevent injuries to the abdominal viscera
B   may cause small bowel injuries
C   do not reduce the incidence of head injuries amongst car
    passengers involved in a road traffic accident
D   protect the cervical spine during sudden acceleration
E   often do not prevent thoracic injuries

146   Indication of a serious intra-abdominal injury in a comatose patient may be gained by
A   abdominal paracentesis
B   the observation of pattern bruising on the abdominal wall
C   falling haemoglobin values
D   the presence of diarrhoea
E   a falling blood pressure

144　A　**True**　Crushing or tearing of the bowel may occur and result in a perforation.

　　B　**True**　Bleeding from a submucosal vessel may produce an intramural haematoma large enough to cause intestinal obstruction.

　　C　**True**　'Stress' ulcers of the stomach and duodenum may follow any hypotensive episode.

　　D　**False**　The signs of peritonitis, or of intra-adominal haemorrhage necessitate urgent laparotomy.

　　E　**False**　The retroperitoneal structures are frequently damaged by trauma to the loins and the pancreas from anterior injuries which crush the pancreas against the vertebral column.

145　A　**False**　Serious injuries to bowel, mesenteric vessels,
　　B　**True**　pancreas and kidney may still occur during sudden deceleration. It should be emphasised that the injuries would have been more serious had a belt not been worn.

　　C　**False**　Seat belts largely prevent dashboard and windscreen head injuries.

　　D　**False**　'Whiplash' injuries to the cervical spine can occur during a sudden acceleration even when seat belts are worn. They may be reduced by the introduction of head rests.

　　E　**False**　Serious thoracic injuries are very uncommon in those wearing seat belts.

146　A　**True**　Aspiration of blood or purulent peritoneal fluid suggests visceral injury.

　　B　**True**　When the pattern of clothing is imprinted on the abdominal wall, it implies that a severe crush injury has occurred.

　　C　**True**　This may denote a splenic or liver rupture.

　　D　**False**　There is no association.

　　E　**True**　A falling blood pressure in the absence of obvious loss of blood or chest trauma in patients with multiple injuries is almost always caused by intra-abdominal problems.

147 Penetrating wounds of the abdomen

A can be adequately explored and their depth determined by a probe

B frequently result in acquired abdominal wall herniae

C may be managed by careful observation, laparotomy being indicated only if signs of peritonitis or blood loss occur

D demand an urgent laparotomy

E can be treated conservatively if the weapon is less than 3 cm long

148 Urinary tract injuries

A are usually accompanied by some degree of haematuria

B require an urgent intravenous pyelogram and possibly a cystogram

C involving the kidney require urgent surgery

D which demonstrate urine extravasating from the bladder are generally managed conservatively

E may accompany crushing injuries to the pelvis

149 Injuries to the urethra

A are usually confined to the male

B are often caused by road traffic accidents

C are readily diagnosed on intravenous pyelography

D require urgent surgical treatment

E usually heal without sequelae

147 A **False** The shuttering and overriding actions of the abdominal wall muscles prevent full exploration with a probe.

  B **False** This is no more common than after laparotomy.

  C **True** If the patient is observed carefully, his vital and abdominal signs being monitored hourly by an

  D **False** experienced clinician, an unnecessary laparotomy may be avoided.

  E **False** Compression of the abdomen wall occurs during penetration, thus allowing short objects to enter the peritoneal cavity and the viscera.

148 A **True** The amount of haematuria does not relate to the degree of damage to the urinary tract.

  B **True** These two investigations will, in most cases, localise the injury, establish whether the patient has two kidneys and determine the function of each.

  C **False** The early management of the injured kidney is, in most cases, by observation.

  D **False** Urgent surgery is indicated once this diagnosis is made.

  E **True** Pelvic fractures are occasionally associated with injuries to the urinary bladder.

149 A **False** Fractures of the pelvis in either sex may result in a

  B **True** torn membranous urethra. In the male the prostate and bladder may then be displaced upwards.

  C **False** Failure to pass urine, after a pelvic injury, should arouse suspicion and, if gentle catheterisation is not possible, urethrograms or laparotomy will be required to establish the diagnosis.

  D **True** Diversion of the urinary stream and restoration of

  E **False** urethral continuity should be undertaken in every case in order to avoid extravasation, periurethral fibrosis and stricture formation.

150 Renal trauma

A   should always be suspected in any patient with abdominal trauma
B   usually presents with haematuria
C   usually requires surgical management
D   always requires an intravenous pyelogram
E   often presents with acute renal failure

151 The spleen

A   is the commonest organ injured in blunt abdominal trauma
B   usually continues to bleed once its capsule is torn and its pulp lacerated
C   either bleeds immediately or not at all after a pulp injury
D   should be removed if there has been a laceration of its capsule
E   has important immunological functions

150 A **True**   The absence of haematuria on microscopic examination of the urine will usually exclude this possibility.
   B **True**   The commonest results of blunt trauma to the kidney
   C **False**   are relatively minor contusions or lacerations to the renal parenchyma. These cause loin pain and overt or microscopic haematuria. Surgery is not necessary except in the rare cases of major lacerations or injuries to the renal pedicle.
   D **True**   This is a most important investigation. Not only may it confirm the suspected injury but it will also present evidence of the presence or absence of the contralateral kidney.
   E **False**   This is rare but may follow severe injury to a solitary kidney or severe bilateral injuries.

151 A **True**   On account of its thin capsule, proximity to the ribs and its relatively mobile nature.
   B **True**   A torn capsule with a pulp laceration is unlikely to
   C **False**   stop bleeding. A pulp laceration lying deep to an intact capsule may produce a subcapsular haematoma which develops over a period of days, weeks or months. Delayed spontaneous haemorrhage will almost certainly ensue. It is advisable to remove any spleen which has any signs of trauma.
   D **False**   Splenectomy should be avoided where oversewing
   E **True**   or limited excision is possible. In children and possibly also in adults, a total splenectomy is followed by an increased risk of dangerous streptococcal infections.

152 Traumatic rupture of the spleen
  A not infrequently presents more than 7 days after the causative injury
  B frequently presents with shoulder tip pain
  C may be diagnosed by paracentesis
  D may, in the absence of hypovolaemia, be treated conservatively
  E may require pneumococcal immunisation

152 A **True**   In 20 per cent of cases the rupture is delayed for up
               to 2 weeks after the injury. This is usually due to a
               delayed rupture of a subcapsular haematoma in the
               peritoneal cavity.
     B **True**   This is usually left sided and indicates the left-sided
               diaphragmatic irritation that is common in this
               condition.
     C **True**   A four quadrant paracentesis through a fine needle is
               valuable in the investigation of any suspected
               abdominal injury. A negative paracentesis does not
               exclude the possibility of a haemoperitoneum but a
               positive aspirate will encourage early laparotomy.
     D **True**   The recognition of the complications of
               immunological defects following splenectomy,
               particularly in children, have led to a more
               conservative approach when hypovolaemia and
               peritonitis are absent. Frequent ultrasound scanning
               may be used to monitor splenic size and the
               presence or absence of perisplenic haematomata.
     E **True**   Splenectomies in children and possibly the elderly
               should be followed by active immunisation against
               pneumococcal meningitis. Some advise long term
               antibiotics also to prevent the increased incidence of
               this infection after splenectomy.

9 The acute abdomen

153 Acute abdominal pain which is
- **A** colicky in nature indicates obstruction of a hollow viscus
- **B** continuous is typical of inflammation
- **C** maximal in the right loin is typical of duodenal ulceration
- **D** in the right upper quadrant accentuated by inspiration is typical of cholecystitis
- **E** in the upper abdomen always indicates intra-abdominal pathology

154 In the acute abdomen, vomiting
- **A** occurring soon after the onset of colicky pain often indicates pathology outside the gastrointestinal tract
- **B** of fluid containing no bile is characteristic of small bowel obstruction
- **C** of faeculent fluid usually indicates a gastrocolic fistula
- **D** is a common early accompaniment of gastroduodenal perforation
- **E** which is projectile and of large volume often indicates an obstruction at the cardia

153 A **True** Ureteric colic arises in the lumbar region and spreads down via the iliac fossa towards the external genitalia; biliary colic will characteristically be maximal in the right upper quadrant; intestinal colic will be referred to the midline anteriorly.

B **True** Whether this arises from infection, haemorrhage or ischaemia.

C **False** Duodenal pain is felt in the epigastrium. Loin pain is usually of renal origin.

D **True** But be aware that diaphragmatic irritation from
E **False** pleural or pulmonary pathology may produce the same kind of pain.

---

154 A **True** Both biliary and renal colic produce 'reflex' vomiting coincident with the pain. This will, however, also occur with a high small bowel obstruction.

B **False** This almost always indicates gastric pathology, particularly pyloric stenosis.

C **False** This is a very rare cause of faeculent vomiting. The usual cause is well-developed lower small bowel obstruction. Bacterial proliferation and decomposition of the stagnant bowel contents causes this faeculent change.

D **False** Vomiting is an uncommon early symptom in this condition.

E **False** These are symptoms of gastric outlet obstruction (pyloric stenosis). Obstruction of the cardia produces dysphagia and regurgitation but no vomiting.

155   Faeculent vomiting

F   A   is commonly seen after upper gastrointestinal tract bleeding
F   B   indicates large bowel obstruction
T   C   indicates bacterial proliferation in the upper intestinal tract
T   D   suggests a gastrocolic fistula
    E   usually presents with a patient who is also hypovolaemic

156   A patient with generalised peritonitis

T   A   usually has an elevated temperature and pulse rate
F   B   characteristically complains of spasmodic severe pain which causes him to be restless
F   C   characteristically vomits
    D   will usually have a rapid and deep respiratory pattern
F   E   may require paracentesis for diagnosis of the condition

157   A perforated duodenal ulcer

F   A   usually lies on the anterior or superior surface of the duodenum
T   B   usually presents with the acute onset of severe back pain
T   C   produces radiological evidence of free gas in the peritoneum in over 90 per cent of the patients
T   D   is usually treated surgically by simple closure of the perforation
?   E   should, if detected within the first 4 hours, be treated by cimetidine or ranitidine

155 A **False**   Small bowel obstruction always results in bacterial
     B **False**   proliferation, and decomposition of the small bowel
     C **True**   contents then occur. The smell and appearance of
                    such vomitus is faeculent. Altered blood is usually
                    darker and less foul smelling. Faeculent vomiting is a
                    late (and relatively infrequent) sign of large bowel
                    obstruction.
     D **False**   In this rare condition, if vomiting occurs then the
                    vomitus may contain faeces. It does not have the
                    homogeneity of faeculent vomiting.
     E **True**   Faeculant vomiting only occurs when intestinal
                    obstruction is well established and fluid shifts have
                    occurred, which, together with decreased fluid intake,
                    reduce the patient to a hypovolaemic state.

156 A **True**   Though these may take a few hours to develop.
     B **False**   The pain is severe, constant and widespread and the
                    patient lies motionless since movement exacerbates
                    the pain.
     C **True**   This is almost constantly present. At first it is reflex in
                    nature and the volume is small but as the effects of
                    the ensuing paralytic ileus develop the vomit
                    increases in volume.
     D **False**   The respiratory movements though rapid are shallow
                    for diaphragmatic and abdominal wall movements
                    increase the pain.
     E **True**   Paracentesis, the withdrawal of 5 to 10 ml of
                    peritoneal fluid by an infraumbilical needle puncture,
                    is occasionally used when the diagnosis is in doubt.

157 A **True**   Penetrating posterior ulcers usually bleed after
                    erosion of the gastroduodenal artery; anterior ulcers
                    perforate rather than bleed.
     B **False**   By far the commonest presentation is the acute onset
                    of severe epigastric pain which rapidly spreads to the
                    whole abdomen.
     C **False**   Less than 75 per cent of perforated ulcers show free
                    gas under the diaphragm on an erect film of the
                    abdomen.
     D **True**   For acute ulcers and small chronic ulcers this is
                    advised. In perforation of large ulcers definitive
                    surgery, i.e. vagotomy and pyloroplasty or partial
                    gastrectomy is usually preferred, provided that
                    peritoneal contamination is neither extensive nor
                    well established.
     E **False**   Only the rare, severely compromised frail patients
                    should be denied surgery.

158 Congenital pyloric stenosis
   A   occurs more commonly in male children
   B   usually presents in the first few days of life
   C   presents with bile-stained vomiting
   D   is usually diagnosed on clinical examination
   E   should usually be treated surgically

159 Acute appendicitis
   A   is most common in the 30 to 40 year age group
   B   characteristically presents with a high temperature
   C   is often associated with painful extension of the right hip
   D   may produce haematuria and pyuria
   E   can be excluded if the patient has diarrhoea

158 A **True** Boys are affected four times as commonly as girls. There is some evidence of a hereditary tendency.

  B **False** The signs of pyloric obstruction usually present after the second week of life. By this time oedema of the pyloric mucosa contributes to the narrowing, produced by the hypertrophied pyloric muscle, to cause obstruction.

  C **False** Projectile vomiting, particularly after feeds, occurs, but this is not bile stained since the obstruction is proximal to the ampulla of Vater.

  D **True** If the abdomen is examined after the infant has been fed, forceful transverse peristaltic waves can usually be seen passing from left to right across the upper abdomen and the abnormal mass of hypertrophied muscle, the 'pyloric tumour', becomes palpable.

  E **True** Surgical treatment is indicated once fluid and electrolyte imbalance has been corrected. Medical management, though often advocated in the past, has not proved to be very successful.

159 A **False** The peak incidence is in the 15 to 25 year age group. It is uncommon in the very young and the very old (but more dangerous and difficult to diagnose).

  B **False** Temperature and pulse are frequently normal in the disease. The temperature rarely exceeds 38°C unless perforation or abscess formation has occurred.

  C **True** The retrocaecal position is the most common and in this position the inflamed appendix may produce spasm of iliopsoas and painful limited extension of the right hip. This is a useful diagnostic sign.

  D **True** Right-sided renal and ureteric colic are frequently confused with appendicitis. The detection of red cells in the urine usually indicates urinary calculi as the cause. However, an inflamed appendix that lies adjacent to the right ureter or bladder may produce urinary signs and symptoms such as haematuria and pyuria.

  E **False** A retro-ileal appendix, or more commonly an appendicitis that presents with a pelvis abscess, will produce diarrhoea.

160 Appendicitis is

A   more common in females
B   distributed evenly throughout the world's population
C   more likely to occur if the appendix is in the retrocaecal position
D   commonly the result of appendicular obstruction
E   frequently recurrent

161 The physical signs of early appendicitis

A   are generally of more diagnostic value than the patient's history
B   usually include muscle guarding in the right iliac fossa
C   usually include a pyrexia above 38.5°C
D   include rectal tenderness
E   usually include a palpable mass in the right iliac fossa

162 Patients with early appendicitis

A   usually present with central abdominal pain
B   rarely present with anorexia
C   have usually vomited on one or two occasions
D   usually complain of similar attacks of pain in the previous few weeks
E   usually have no premonitory signs or symptoms.

160 A **False** The incidence is the same in both sexes.
     B **False** The disease is uncommon in the underdeveloped
                   countries of the Third World.
     C **False** Though this is the commonest position of the
                   appendix, it carries no increased risk of appendicitis.
     D **True**   Appendicitis follows obstruction of the appendicular
                   lumen due either to lymphoid hyperplasia (which is
                   particularly common in children), a faecolith (which
                   is found in almost half the cases), or, rarely, to a
                   tumour or stricture.
     E **False** Though some cases will resolve spontaneously and
                   occur again this is infrequently seen.

161 A **False** Usually the reverse is true.
     B **True**   This resistance to palpation is a guide to the severity
                   of the inflammation and it progresses to involuntary
                   rigidity.
     C **False** A milder pyrexia is common. High fever is
                   uncommon until perforation or abscess formation
                   occurs.
     D **True**   A rectal examination should always be performed.
                   Rectal tenderness in the pouch of Douglas may
                   provide the only positive evidence of appendicitis
                   when the inflamed organ lies in the pelvis, but is not
                   invariably present.
     E **False** This sign produced by a periappendicular abscess is
                   not invariably present. It is only usually found in
                   cases undiagnosed for several days.

162 A **True**   This is felt most severely in the umbilical region. In a
                   few cases such a history is not obtained.
     B **False** Anorexia is almost always noted in patients with
                   appendicitis.
     C **True**   This follows the abdominal pain and may be reflex in
                   nature.
     D **False** Though recurrent appendicitis occasionally occurs it
                   is rare. A history of previous abdominal pain should
                   alert the clinician to think of other causes of the
                   abdominal pain.
     E **True**   There are usually no premonitory signs or
                   symptoms.

163   Investigation of a case of acute appendicitis

A will usually reveal a polymorphonuclear leucocytosis
B often shows microscopic haematuria
C usually reveals haemoconcentration
D often reveals fluid levels in the right iliac fossa on an erect radiograph of the abdomen
E will show faecal occult blood tests to be positive

164   Likely differential diagnoses in a young woman with appendicitis include

A ovulatory pain
B ruptured ectopic pregnancy
C colonic diverticulitis
D caecal carcinoma
E torted ovarian cyst

165   Appendicectomy should be undertaken

A after laparotomy reveals a diagnosis of mesenteric adenitis
B immediately in adult patients with an appendix abscess
C in patients with a gangrenous appendix
D in patients with chronic appendicitis
E if its inflammation is the result of neighbouring Crohn's disease

166   Obstruction of the lumen of the appendix may lead to

A mucosal ulceration
B gangrenous appendicitis
C a perforated appendix
D intussusception of the appendix
E atrophy in the appendix

163 A **True**   Too much emphasis should not be placed on
     B **True**   laboratory tests for their discriminatory value is
                   slight.
     C **False** Though there is usually a leucocytosis this is not
                   constant. About one-quarter of patients will show
                   leucocytes or red cells in the urine but there is rarely
                   a raised haematocrit in the early case.
     D **False** Abdominal radiology is not often helpful. When there
                   is radiological evidence of appendicitis (such as the
                   absence of small bowel gas in the right iliac fossa,
                   gas under the diaphragm or a scoliosis concave to
                   the right), the diagnosis is usually clinically obvious.
     E **False** Appendicitis is not associated with bleeding into the
                   bowel lumen.

164 A **True**   Midcycle ovulatory pain last for only a few hours.
     B **True**   Often there is a history of a missed menstruation and
                   the presence of a tender tubal mass is noted on
                   pelvic examination.
     C **False** Colonic diverticulitis and caecal cancer may mimic
     D **False** appendicitis, but it is extremely uncommon for these
                   to occur in this age group.
     E **True**   But torsion of the ovarian cyst usually has a more
                   sudden and severe onset with right iliac fossa pain
                   from the outset.

165 A **True**   The procedure is prophylactic and carries little
                   additional morbidity and mortality.
     B **False** It is usually wisest to surgically drain the abscess and
                   unless the appendix can be removed easily it should
                   be left for an interval appendicectomy some 2
                   months later.
     C **True**   In all cases.
     D **True**   This disputed condition occurs but is not common.
     E **True**   Crohn's ileitis may mimic appendicitis. If the
                   appendix is inflamed it should be removed.

166 A **True**   Luminal obstruction leads to oedema and distension
     B **True**   of the distal appendix, mucosal ulcers appear and as
     C **True**   the distension increases the venous drainage and
                   arterial supply are impeded and gangrenous
                   perforation may occur. Peritonitis may then follow
                   and the mortality rises.
     D **False** These are not related to appendicular obstruction.
     E **False**

167   In the differential diagnosis of appendicitis in an infant it is important to consider
A   ileo-ileal intussusception
B   basal pneumonia
C   Henoch–Schoenlein purpura
D   torsion of an ovarian cyst
E   testicular torsion

168   Acute non-specific mesenteric lymphadenitis
A   is commonest between 5 and 12 years of age
B   is usually associated with an upper respiratory tract infection
C   is usually associated with cervical lymphadenopathy
D   is characterised by enlarged mesenteric lymph nodes which are infected by Gram-negative organisms
E   should be treated by antibiotics

169   Abdominal distension in mechanical intestinal obstruction is produced in part by
A   swallowed air
B   carbon dioxide produced in the bowel
C   increased intestinal secretions proximal to the obstruction
D   decreased intestinal absorption proximal to the obstruction
E   peritoneal exudate

167 A **True**   Screaming and intermittent abdominal colic, a short
                    history of melaena and palpation of a sausage-
                    shaped mass are classical signs of childhood
                    intussusception. However, nausea and abdominal
                    distension are often the only symptoms.
     B **True**   Diaphragmatic pleurisy may produce referred pain in
                    the lower abdomen.
     C **True**   A haematoma of the small bowel wall may mimic
                    appendicitis but the presence of a purpuric rash and
                    joint pains should arouse suspicion of
                    Henoch–Schoenlein purpura.
     D **False** This is very uncommon before puberty.
     E **False** This is rare in infancy, though when it occurs the pain
                    may be indicated to lie in the right iliac fossa.

168 A **True**   Although it is less common than appendicitis in this
                    age group.
     B **True**   This is commonly coexistent with, or precedes the
                    vague, colicky, lower abdominal pain by a few days.
     C **True**   There is frequently pharyngeal injection. Examination
                    of the abdomen reveals tenderness which is higher,
                    more medial and more variable in position than
                    appendicitis. The leucocyte count is moderately
                    raised to 12 000 to 15 000/mm^3 (12 000 to 15 000/μl).
     D **False** Although mesenteric lymph nodes enlargement is
                    characteristically present, cultures of the nodes are
                    usually sterile.
     E **False** The condition is short lived, lasting no more than 3 to
                    5 days. It is generally a viral condition and antibiotics
                    are not indicated in treatment.

169 A **True**   Nitrogen is not readily absorbed by the intestine,
                    thus more than 70 per cent of the accumulated gas
                    comes from swallowed air.
     B **False** Though large quantities of carbon dioxide are
                    produced in the bowel, accumulation does not occur
                    because this gas is readily absorbed.
     C **True**   In the distended bowel there is a gross disturbance of
     D **True**   the usual absorption/secretion activities of the
                    intestinal mucosa. Both increased secretion and
                    decreased absorption of fluid have been shown to
                    occur in a distended bowel proximal to an
                    obstruction.
     E **False** Though there is always an excessive amount of
                    peritoneal fluid in these patients, the excess is not
                    sufficient to contribute to the distension.

170   The level of intestinal obstruction can be determined by
   A   questioning the patient
   B   examining the patient
   C   radiological examination of the patient
   D   repeated measurements of the patient's girth
   E   radiological examination by contrast enema

171   Acute small bowel obstruction
   A   is commonly caused by postoperative adhesions
   B   accompanied by the signs of peritonitis, suggests bowel strangulation
   C   is often associated with a raised serum amylase
   D   generally produces abdominal distension within 2 to 3 hours of onset
   E   may exist with no disturbance of defaecation

170 A **True**   In high small bowel obstruction vomiting occurs
soon after the onset of pain whereas in large bowel
obstruction vomiting appears much later if at all.
Small bowel colic is felt in the central abdomen;
large bowel colic in the suprapubic region.
Constipation is an early symptom in large bowel
obstruction.

   B **True**   In large bowel obstruction distension is greater and
tends to be most marked in the flanks. The distension
of small bowel obstruction is central abdominal.

   C **True**   In small bowel obstruction there is very little gas in
the colon. Colonic distension can usually be
distinguished from small bowel distension by
haustral markings which occupy only part of the
transverse diameter of the bowel. In distended small
bowel, mucosal folds, the valvulae conniventes, can
be seen traversing the whole diameter.

   D **False**   Except in high small bowel obstruction, progressive
increase in the patient's abdominal girth is a feature
of all types of intestinal obstruction.

   E **True**   The presence and situation of a large bowel
obstruction is frequently confirmed by a water-
soluble contrast enema. This examination also helps
to establish whether or not a colonic pseudo-
obstruction is present.

171 A **True**   Adhesions and exernal herniae are the two
commonest causes. A careful inspection for surgical
scars and of the hernial orifices must therefore be
routine.

   B **True**   A rising temperature and pulse rate and local
abdominal tenderness and rigidity, all indicate that
strangulation is developing. Operative treatment is
then an urgent necessity.

   C **True**   The serum amylase is frequently raised to twice
normal values but should not be confused with the
very high values usually seen in the initial stages of
acute pancreatitis.

   D **False**   Central abdominal distension usually appears after
12 to 24 hours and may be absent in high small
bowel obstruction.

   E **True**   Total constipation is a late feature of small bowel
obstruction.

172   In the treatment of intestinal obstruction
A   nasogastric suction should be instituted preoperatively
B   intravenous fluid replacement is essential
C   abdominal girth measurements allow one to decide when surgical intervention is required
D   immediate surgery is essential
E   surgery should be restricted to those cases where strangulation is diagnosed

173   Emergency treatment of a mechanical obstruction of the large bowel may include
A   enemata
B   radiological examination by contrast enema
C   exteriorisation of the lesion with a colostomy
D   a transverse colostomy
E   an ileo-transverse colostomy

172 A **True**   Aspiration via a nasogastric tube, though having little
     B **True**   effect on the distended bowel, minimises further
                    distension by removing swallowed air. It also
                    reduces the risk of aspiration of vomit. All patients
                    with intestinal obstruction will have abnormal fluid
                    and electrolyte losses – these must be made good by
                    the intravenous administration of isotonic saline,
                    often with potassium supplements.
     C **False**   Measurement of abdominal girth is not only
                    imprecise but irrelevant to the pathological processes
                    that are occurring.
     D **False**   Although in many cases the most appropriate
                    treatment is surgical relief of the obstruction, this
                    should not be performed until careful attention has
                    been paid to correcting fluid and electrolyte
                    deficiencies and nasogastric suction has been
                    instituted.
     E **False**   Strangulation is a serious complication adding
                    peritonitis to the pathophysiology of intestinal
                    obstruction. This is reflected in high mortality rates
                    and therefore surgery should be undertaken before
                    this complication develops.

173 A **True**   Faecal impaction is a cause of large bowel
                    obstruction in the elderly. It may be effectively
                    treated by enemata though disimpaction under
                    general anaesthetic is frequently necessary.
     B **True**   Not all large bowel obstructions are mechanical. A
                    considerable proportion in the elderly are the result
                    of atony of the large bowel, whose causes are not
                    well understood. These cases of 'pseudo-
                    obstruction', which do not require surgery, can be
                    distinguished in this way.
     C **False**   This is no longer a procedure that is advocated.
     D **True**   It is usually unsafe to attempt resection of the
     E **True**   obstructing lesion with primary anastomosis. The
                    majority of cases are managed in the first instance by
                    these simpler methods which permit safe
                    decompression of the proximal bowel.

174   Strangulation of the bowel

  A   commonly complicates closed loop obstruction
  B   is difficult to distinguish from simple intestinal obstruction
  C   is accompanied by bleeding into the affected bowel
  D   frequently causes peritonitis
  E   may result in Gram-negative septicaemia

175   Small bowel obstruction often results in

  A   hyperkalaemia
  B   metabolic alkalosis
  C   oliguria
  D   hypovolaemia
  E   pancreatitis

176   Large bowel obstruction

  A   is most commonly caused by diverticular disease of the colon
  B   has its maximum incidence before the age of 50 years
  C   frequently presents with nausea and vomiting
  D   usually heralds its onset with constant suprapubic pain
  E   may result in the grossest abdominal distension

174 A **True**   When the bowel lumen is closed at two points along its length the raised intraluminal pressure results in impairment of the blood supply to the affected loop and strangulation frequently occurs.
     B **False**   Strangulation should be suspected in any patient with intestinal obstruction who demonstrates signs of local or generalised peritonitis.
     C **True**   Blood and plasma are lost from the strangulated portion and trapped in it following venous obstruction and capillary leakage. As an approximate guide, one litre of blood may be lost per metre of strangulated bowel.
     D **True**   The ischaemic segment of bowel is permeable to the
     E **True**   increased number of bacteria and their toxins. This infected fluid produces peritonitis and its absorption into the general circulation can cause cardiovascular collapse.

175 A **False**   Potassium is lost in intestinal secretions, in vomiting
     B **True**   and in abnormal renal losses which follow attempts to conserve hydrogen ions in the metabolic alkalosis that accompanies proximal small bowel obstruction.
     C **True**   Dehydration rapidly develops due to loss of fluid into
     D **True**   the distended bowel, diminished fluid intake and vomiting. Haemoconcentration, hypovolaemia and oliguria thus rapidly appear.
     E **False**   This is not related.

176 A **False**   Colonic cancer is the most common cause, followed by diverticular disease and sigmoid volvulus. Most of the obstructing cancers are in the descending and sigmoid colon.
     B **False**   This is a disease of the elderly.
     C **False**   These symptoms are usually absent until the late stages of the disease, particularly when the ileocaecal valve is competent.
     D **False**   The visceral pain produced is vague but colicky and felt in the lower abdomen.
     E **True**   The distension is always greater than that produced by small bowel obstruction and, when volvulus of the sigmoid colon or caecum occurs, massive distension will occur.

177 Patients with acute colonic diverticulitis
    A often give a history of recent lower abdominal colic
    B often present with a pyrexia
    C can be frequently diagnosed on sigmoidoscopic appearances
    D frequently develop faecal peritonitis
    E can generally be treated successfully with antibiotics and supportive therapy

178 Acute pancreatitis frequently
    A is accompanied by hypercalcaemia
    B produces paralytic ileus
    C is associated with a pleural effusion
    D produces pyloric stenosis
    E produces hypoxaemia

177 A **True** These symptoms of diverticular disease frequently precede the acute attack.
    B **True** Temperatures of 38°C and above may indicate the presence of a pericolic abscess.
    C **False** Though oedema of the rectosigmoid junction may occasionally be seen, the more inaccessible pelvic colon is the site of the pathology, and out of reach of the sigmoidoscope.
    D **False** Rupture of a pericolic abscess may lead to generalised peritonitis. This complication, which carries a high mortality, is rare. The inflammation more frequently localises as a pericolic abscess.
    E **True** Only a small number of patients fail to respond to these medical measures.

---

178 A **False** Hypocalcaemia is a frequent complication occurring within a few days of the onset. Though it is frequently stated to be a consequence of saponification of retroperitoneal fat, this is almost certainly a too facile explanation and the true cause is still unknown.
    B **True** Even mild attacks generally produce a segmental ileus of the overlying jejunal loops. The distended bowel in the upper abdomen produces characteristic radiological appearances.
    C **True** Most commonly a left-sided effusion, due to subdiaphragmatic inflammation.
    D **False** However, there is frequently distortion of the duodenal loop on a barium meal.
    E **True** Pancreatitis produces widespread systemic effects because of the 'toxic broth' that circulates. The aveolar membranes, like the glomeruli, are affected. Hypoxaemia and oliguria are frequent consequences that must be sought for and corrected.

179 Acute pancreatitis
  A is frequently associated with gallstones
  B often simulates a perforated peptic ulcer in its presentation
  C often presents with the signs of hypovolaemia
  D can readily be distinguished from other causes of acute
       abdominal pain by the presence of a raised serum amylase
  E frequently has a raised concentration of urinary amylase

180 The treatment of acute pancreatitis
  A is largely nonspecific and supportive
  B should include a laparotomy in the majority of cases
  C should routinely include the administration of calcium
  D should routinely include the administration of antibiotics
  E is more effective when peritoneal lavage is included

179 A **True**   Gallstones are present in the majority of cases. It is
                    thought that biliary calculi obstruct either the
                    pancreatic duct or its common junction with the bile
                    duct at the ampulla. Alcohol and viral diseases
                    account for most of the remaining cases.
     B **True**   The disease varies in severity and the epigastric pain
                    may be as severe as that of a perforated peptic ulcer.
                    It commonly radiates to the back and then must be
                    distinguished from a ruptured or dissecting aortic
                    aneurysm.
     C **True**   In a severe attack there is considerable
                    retroperitoneal inflammation and sequestration of
                    fluid which results in hypovolaemia and shock.
     D **False** Although in most cases the serum amylase rises
                    within 8 hours of the onset and remains elevated for
                    2 to 3 days only a rise of approximately four times
                    the normal value will certainly distinguish
                    pancreatitis from the other causes of
                    hyperamylasaemia, viz. gallstones, perforated peptic
                    ulcer, small bowel obstruction and mesenteric
                    thrombosis.
     E **True**   There is a more constant rise in urinary amylase
                    values in pancreatitis than in the above conditions.

180 A **True**   Hypovolaemia should be corrected, continuous
                    nasogastric suction will relieve distension and reduce
                    pancreatic secretion. Pain relief can usually be
                    achieved with pethidine, oxygen will counteract the
                    hypoxia of severe cases and intravenous fluids the
                    tendency towards prerenal failure.
     B **False** Most cases will improve on the above therapy but
                    laparotomy is advised if the patient is deteriorating
                    or if a fever or abdominal mass appears. Usually
                    removal of the necrotic tissue and drainage of the
                    area is all that can be undertaken.
     C **False** It should only be given in those patients who have
                    clinical or biochemical evidence of hypocalcaemia.
     D **False** Antibiotics are essential in the treatment of any
                    infective complications but their prophylactic use is
                    not beneficial.
     E **False** Early reports of its action were enthusiastic but
                    careful studies have subsequently shown no benefit.

181 Childhood intussusception

A usually presents during the first year of life
B is frequently caused by congenital gastrointestinal tract abnormalities
C is frequently ileocolic
D can usually be diagnosed without radiological examination of the abdomen
E rarely requires surgical treatment

182 Meconium ileus

A is the presenting feature in the majority of patients with cystic fibrosis
B may occur at any time in the first year of life
C is associated with achlorhydria
D presents with a distended abdomen and bilious vomiting
E may be effectively treated with acetylcysteine

183 Neonatal duodenal obstruction

A may be associated with Down's syndrome
B is more frequently found in premature infants
C typically presents with gross abdominal distension
D usually presents with vomiting of bile-stained fluid
E requires urgent surgical treatment

181 A **True**   The average age of presentation is gradually becoming younger.
     B **False** The cause is obscure. It is suggested lymphatic
     C **True**   hyperplasia secondary to virus infections or a change in the infant's diet on weaning, may produce a submucosal swelling in the intestinal wall which initiates the intussusception.
     D **True**   Sudden colicky pain, often with the passage of bloody stools, suggests the diagnosis – the palpation of a sausage-shaped mass in the right upper quadrant is confirmatory, but this is not always present.
     E **False** Providing no signs of intestinal strangulation exist, *gentle* reduction by means of a barium enema may be attempted under fluoroscopic control. The majority of patients, however, require surgical intervention.

182 A **False** Only about 10 per cent of patients with cystic fibrosis have meconium ileus.
     B **False** It is a disease of neonates.
     C **False** No abnormalities of gastric secretion occur in this syndrome. There is an associated deficiency of pancreatic function.
     D **True**   Distal ileal obstruction occurs due to abnormally viscous meconium.
     E **True**   This obstruction must usually be relieved surgically or, in mild cases, by the detergent action of orally administered acetylcysteine or Gastrografin, a hypertonic contrast medium.

183 A **True**   More than 20 per cent of such infants will also have Down's syndrome.
     B **False** There is not an increased frequency in premature infants.
     C **False** The obstruction is high and so abdominal distension is usually absent.
     D **True**   Vomiting is frequent, and usually contains bile since the obstruction is usually distal to the ampulla of Vater.
     E **True**   The congenital stricture can be relieved by no other means.

184 Acute gastric dilatation
- A may follow spinal injuries
- B rarely follows abdominal surgery
- C may cause dehydration and hypovolaemia
- D may cause haemorrhagic ulceration
- E requires urgent surgical treatment

185 Acute superior mesenteric artery occlusion
- A characteristically presents with sudden pain and tenderness of increasing intensity
- B is frequently due to embolism
- C is frequently accompanied by overt or occult blood loss in the stools
- D frequently produces peritonitis
- E can usually be diagnosed on plain abdominal radiographs

186 A ruptured ectopic pregnancy
- A usually occurs in the first month of pregnancy
- B usually presents with severe lower abdominal pain
- C frequently presents with hypovolaemic shock
- D can usually be diagnosed by pelvic examination
- E may demonstrate a lower abdominal mass

184 A **True**   Although the mechanism is not known, the
    B **False**   commonest cause in Britain is thought to be due to
                  inadequate nasogastric drainage after abdominal
                  surgery.
    C **True**   There is gastric hypersecretion. Vomiting and
                  diminished fluid intake produce dehydration and
                  hypovolaemia frequently follows.
    D **True**   The vomitus may be bloodstained. Untreated cases
                  have been followed by spontaneous rupture of the
                  stomach.
    E **False**   Effective nasogastric suction is all that is required. All
                  attempts at surgical drainage have been disastrous.

185 A **True**   The pain is often more severe than the abdominal
                  tenderness suggests.
    B **True**   Though thrombosis complicating atherosclerosis is
                  also common.
    C **True**   Intestinal blood loss is almost invariably present and
                  results from haemorrhagic infarction of the bowel
                  mucosa.
    D **True**   Ischaemia of the bowel leads to the bacteria of the
                  bowel 'leaking' into the peritoneal cavity with
                  catastrophic results.
    E **False**   Radiographs are usually unhelpful. Occasionally
                  intrahepatic gas is seen as the ominous result of gas-
                  forming organisms ascending via the portal vein to
                  the liver.

186 A **False**   Rupture usually occurs between the sixth and twelfth
                  weeks of pregnancy. There is often a history of a
                  missed or scanty menstrual period.
    B **True**   This is associated with vomiting and a desire to
                  defaecate.
    C **True**   A large proportion of patients with this life-
                  threatening condition suffer a rapid and severe blood
                  loss.
    D **True**   A tender cervix and a boggy mass in the vaginal
                  fornices are usually palpable.
    E **True**   Large tubal masses may be palpable abdominally.

187 Acute salpingitis

A   usually occurs in the first month of pregnancy
B   is frequently associated with vomiting
C   often presents with vaginal discharge
D   presents with uterine tenderness
E   is usually caused by *Staphylococcus aureus*

188 A ruptured ovarian cyst

A   most frequently occurs premenstrually
B   is more common in those on oral contraceptives
C   may cause peritonitis
D   most commonly occurs in young women
E   requires no surgical treatment

189 Biliary colic typically

A   occurs 3 to 4 hours after meals
B   lasts 5 to 20 minutes
C   radiates from the upper abdomen to the right subscapular
    region
D   is made worse by deep inspiration
E   is followed by jaundice

187   A   **False**   The majority of cases are post-abortal or puerperal.
      B   **True**   Other gastrointestinal disturbances are unusual.
      C   **False**   This is not a marked feature except in those rare
                      cases which have followed uterine infections.
      D   **True**   Vaginal examination will reveal this, together with a
                      tender cervix and tenderness in one or other vaginal
                      fornices.
      E   **False**   Gram-negative organisms and *Bacteroides* are the
                      usual organisms.

188   A   **False**   Follicular cyst rupture is the commonest and occurs
                      mid-menstrually. More rarely a luteal cyst may
                      rupture and this will occur premenstrually.
      B   **False**   No such association has been shown.
      C   **True**   Bleeding from the cyst frequently occurs. This causes
                      haemoperitoneum and local peritonitis.
      D   **True**
      E   **False**   Very frequently laparotomy is required to exclude
                      appendicitis. Surgical treatment of the cyst and
                      haemostasis are necessary in a proportion of
                      patients.

189   A   **False**   The patient usually gives a past history of dyspepsia,
      B   **False**   viz. postprandial flatulence, nausea and epigastric
                      pain. Biliary colic usually occurs soon after a meal
                      and lasts at least 3 to 4 hours and often a day or
                      more.
      C   **True**   The pain is initially felt in the epigastrium or right
                      hypochondrium and later radiates to the back or right
                      subscapular region.
      D   **True**   It is accentuated by deep breathing.
      E   **False**   Biliary colic emanates from gallbladder contractions
                      and there is usually no associated obstruction of the
                      common bile duct.

10 Stomach, duodenum and small intestine

190 Benign gastric ulcers
A occur in the same age group as duodenal ulcers
B are more common in males than females
C are more common in the upper social classes
D produce epigastric pain after eating food
E are occasionally premalignant

191 Uncomplicated benign gastric ulcers
A occur most commonly on the greater curve of the stomach
B should initially be treated medically
C commonly recur after medical treatment
D require endoscopic surveillance during treatment
E should receive surgical treatment if healing has not occurred after 8 weeks of medical treatment

190 A **False** They are commoner in older people. The peak incidence for duodenal ulcers is around 30 years whereas gastric ulcers are most common around 50 years of age.
B **True** The disease is twice as common in men.
C **False** There is an increased incidence in the lower social classes.
D **True** The pain of gastric ulceration is characteristically felt in the epigastrium and is made worse by eating or drinking strong alcoholic beverages.
E **False** Benign gastric ulcers do not become malignant but ulcerating gastric cancers may be misdiagnosed as benign ulcers. All gastric ulcers require careful endoscopic surveillance and repeated multiple biopsies to lessen this risk of misdiagnosis.

191 A **False** The commonest site is on the lesser curve, particularly around the incisura angularis.
B **True** Particularly if gastroscopy and endoscopic biopsy indicate that the ulcer is benign.
C **True** Recurrence rates of as high as 50 per cent have been reported after intensive medical management with antacids or H₂ blockade.
D **True** Endoscopy is far more reliable than radiology when following the course of the ulcer. It also offers the facilities for biopsy – an essential part of management.
E **True** If gastroscopic or radiological evidence of healing has not occurred at the end of this period, surgical treatment (usually as Billroth 1 partial gastrectomy with excision of the ulcer) should be undertaken. These patients are at risk from haemorrhage or perforation. Awareness of the fact that approximately 5 per cent of indolent non-healing benign ulcers may be ulcerating cancers masquerading in a benign guise gives further justification to this 'aggressive' approach to treatment.

192 Gastric cancer is
   A   more common in males than females
   B   more common in the higher social classes
   C   increasing in frequency in the United Kingdom
   D   frequently determined by genetic factors
   E   of increased frequency in those patients with atrophic
       gastritis

193 Gastric cancer
   A   is most common in the fundus of the stomach
   B   is most commonly a squamous cell carcinoma
   C   frequently metastasises via the bloodstream
   D   is most frequently an ulcerating lesion
   E   is frequently multifocal

192 A **True**   Throughout the world the incidence in males is
                   approximately twice that of females.
     B **False** Studies from Scandinavia, Japan, USA and the UK all
                   indicate an increased incidence in the lower social
                   classes.
     C **False** The incidence is decreasing slightly in the UK as in
                   the rest of the world. This is most striking in the USA
                   where incidence rates in the 1980s were one-quarter
                   those in the 1930s.
     D **False** Studies of migrants reveal a dominant role for
                   environmental, rather than genetic, factors.
     E **True**   Screening of patients with atrophic gastritis, for
                   instance in patients with pernicious anaemia, reveals
                   an incidence of stomach cancer of 5 to 10 per cent
                   during 10 years' surveillance.

193 A **False** Most cancers are situated around the prepyloric and
                   antral regions, especially along the lesser curve.
     B **False** Almost all gastric carcinomas are adenocarcinomas.
     C **True**   It spreads via the portal blood to produce liver
                   metastases. Systemic blood spread is less common.
                   In addition it may spread by lymphatic permeation,
                   direct extension to neighbouring structures and
                   transcoelomically to produce peritoneal and ovarian
                   metastases.
     D **False** Ulcerating cancers form the minority. The majority
                   have a polypoid form or are diffusely infiltrating
                   (linitis plastica).
     E **True**   Between 10 and 15 per cent of gastric cancers are
                   multifocal.

194 There is an association of gastric cancer with
   A achlorhydria of the stomach
   B atrophic gastritis
   C adenomatous gastric polyps
   D duodenal ulceration
   E a history of gastric cancer in first degree relatives

195 A patient with the signs and symptoms of gastric cancer
   A may simulate those of a benign gastric ulcer
   B may present with a hard palpable left supraclavicular node
   C requires investigation by a barium meal examination
   D requires investigation by a gastroscopic examination even
       when the barium meal is normal
   E should be given therapeutic treatment with H_2 blockers

194 A **True**   A three- to fourfold increase in incidence has frequently been observed in achlorhydric patients with pernicious anaemia. The majority of patients with gastric cancer have achlorhydria or hypochlorhydria.

  B **True**   Long term follow-up of patients with atrophic gastritis has revealed that a higher than expected incidence of gastric cancer is present.

  C **True**   Gastric polyps are rare but approximately 20 per cent of them are malignant, especially those which are greater than 2 cm in diameter.

  D **False**   There is no association. Indeed gastric cancer is extremely uncommon in patients with active duodenal ulceration.

  E **True**   Genetic factors are present, but less dominant than environmental ones. There is a two- to fourfold increase in incidence amongst those with first degree relatives affected with gastric cancer.

195 A **True**   Pain is the commonest first symptom and may mimic that of gastric or duodenal ulceration. It thus demands a full investigation when appearing in any patient over the age of 50 years.

  B **False**   Neoplastic involvement of Virchow's node is a sign of widespread incurable malignancy originating in the upper gastrointestinal tract.

  C **True**   The diagnostic accuracy of a barium meal for
  D **True**   stomach cancer is approximately 80 per cent. For this reason a negative barium meal in a patient suspected of stomach cancer should be followed by a gastroscopic examination.

  E **False** H_2 blockers, such as cimetidine or ranitidine, will frequently relieve dyspeptic symptoms even when these have a neoplastic cause. Dyspepsia occurring above the age of 50 years is an indication for early endoscopic investigation.

196 Surgical treatment of gastric cancer
   A should preferably be by a total gastrectomy
   B gives overall 5-year survival figures of 5 to 10 per cent
   C includes excision of the tumour as a palliative measure
   D should be advised for all diagnosed cases
   E is not more effective when it includes radical excision of the
      regional lymph nodes

197 Duodenal diverticulae
   A most commonly arise from the concavity of the second part
   B are frequently the site of infection, haemorrhage or
      ulceration
   C may be associated with obstructive jaundice
   D may follow a severe case of pancreatitis
   E are usually asymptomatic

198 Duodenal ulcers
   A have an equal incidence in both sexes
   B have a clinical course characterised by long periods of
      remission of symptoms
   C are characterised by postprandial pain
   D occur most commonly in the duodenal cap
   E have a premalignant potential

196 A **False**   The use of total gastrectomy to treat stomach cancer does not improve the survival figures except in the case of carcinomas of the cardia.
    B **True**   Surgical series do report higher 5-year survival in those patients having gastrectomies but the resectability rate is rarely higher than 50 per cent. The 5-year survival rate for patients who had no lymph node metastases at the time of operation is over 40 per cent.
    C **True**   Excision is usually more effective palliation than bypass procedures.
    D **False**   At least 20 per cent of the patients will present with signs of incurable disease, such as a malignant liver enlargement, malignant ascites or a palpable left supraclavicular node. Only necessary palliation should be attempted in these cases.
    E **False**   An attempted curative resection achieves a much better result when it includes radical en bloc resection of the regional lymph nodes.

197 A **True**   A few may also arise from the third part.
    B **False**   They are only very rarely associated with any
    C **False**   pathology. Though narrow necked diverticulitis is
    D **False**   uncommon and no cases of associated obstructive jaundice have been reported, there are only about 30 cases of rupture of these diverticulae reported; therefore elective surgical excision is not advised.
    E **False**   The majority are congenital and not the cause of any symptoms.

198 A **False**   They are four to five times more common in males.
    B **True**   This 'periodicity' of the symptoms, wherein remissions alternate with exacerbations lasting from 1 week to many months, is characteristic.
    C **False**   The epigastric pain generally appears several hours after eating, and thus quite commonly awakes the patient from sleep. It is frequently relieved by food.
    D **True**   95 per cent of ulcers are in the first 1.5 cm of the duodenum (the duodenal cap).
    E **False**   Duodenal cancer is very uncommon and it and stomach cancer are almost unknown in association.

199   The treatment of duodenal ulcers in young patients
   A   can include antacids
   B   can include a strict dietary regime
   C   should include anticholinergic drugs
   D   demands the long term use of H_2 blockers, such as cimetidine or ranitidine
   E   should be by early surgery

200   Chronic duodenal ulcers may be treated by
   A   histamine H_2-receptor antagonists
   B   sub-total gastrectomy
   C   vagotomy and gastric drainage
   D   highly selective vagotomy (HSV)
   E   non-steroidal anti-inflammatory drugs (NSAIDs)

199 A **True** Antacids achieve symptomatic relief by increasing the intragastric pH. However, as this effect does not last longer than 1 hour, frequent administration is necessary.

   B **False** Some patients recognise foods that cause exacerbations of pain and avoid them. However, in general, dietary control has no part to play in the management of these ulcers.

   C **False** To be effective in reducing acid output the drugs must be given in doses large enough to be associated with a high incidence of unpleasant side-effects. For this reason they are not generally recommended.

   D **False** H_2 blockers are best used to treat exacerbation of symptoms. Their long term use over many years has not yet been fully validated. Few clinicians would recommend their daily, life long use to a young patient.

   E **False** Duodenal ulcers are extremely common but of very varying severity. Many symptoms are short lived and of minor consequence. The usual indications for surgery are severe and protracted discomfort or complications.

---

200 A **True** A patient with a chronic history, i.e. two or more attacks, will always have the tendency to ulceration.

   B **True** Effective long term reduction in acid secretion can be
   C **True** achieved by an H_2-antagonist or by any of these
   D **True** operations. Long term medical treatment is often indicated in the elderly patient. All the operations mentioned aid ulcer healing and are used in that minority of patients not treated more appropriately by long term medication. Though subtotal gastrectomy has a low recurrent ulcer rate (2 to 3 per cent) its mortality (2 per cent) and high incidence of side effects compare unfavourably with vagotomy and drainage and HSV. The latter two operations account for the majority of operations on duodenal ulcer patients at present.

   E **False** NSAIDs, though valuable in achieving symptomatic relief from arthritis, should be used cautiously if at all in patients with known gastroduodenal ulceration. They are a potent and frequent cause of gastroduodenal ulceration and contribute to these complications.

201 Acute haemorrhage from the upper gastrointestinal tract

A   requires an urgent barium meal examination
B   requires an urgent gastroscopy
C   should be treated surgically as soon as the diagnosis is made
D   indicates the presence of a chronic duodenal ulcer
E   should be treated with H$_2$ blockade

202 Perforated duodenal ulcers

A   usually have an insidious clinical onset
B   must be treated surgically
C   are common in the elderly
D   are heralded by worsening dyspepsia
E   have a high mortality (more than 5 per cent)

201 A **False**   Diagnosis of the source of the haemorrhage should
     B **True**   be sought urgently in order that rational treatment
                    may be instituted. A barium meal will not identify the
                    source of the bleeding, oesophagogastroscopy will.
     C **False**   The majority of haemorrhages from duodenal ulcers
                    do not require urgent surgery. Surgery is indicated
                    only in peptic disease and when the estimated blood
                    loss is more than 1.5 litres, or when there is a second
                    major haemorrhage within a few days of the first.
                    Since old people withstand hypovolaemia poorly,
                    surgery should be undertaken at an earlier stage in
                    this group.
     D **False**   Erosions, Mallory–Weiss tears and varices, though
                    less common than peptic ulcer, contribute to acute
                    gastrointestinal bleeding problems.
     E **False**   There is no evidence that H_2 blockade either stops
                    bleeding or decreases the incidence of rebleeding.

202 A **False**   The presentation is almost always dramatic with the
                    sudden appearance of worsening epigastric pain.
     B **False**   It is reasonable, in the very frail, to try conservative
                    management with nasogastric aspiration,
                    intravenous fluids and antibiotics, provided the
                    patient is not shocked, and a Gastrografin meal
                    suggests that the perforation is sealed off.
     C **True**   Modern medical treatment has reduced the rate of
                    perforation in younger patients, but the elderly
                    patient is now suffering more perforations, possibly
                    as a result of increased use of ulcerogenic non-
                    steroidal anti-inflammatory drugs.
     D **False**   This is a rare presentation and often the perforation
                    is the first recorded symptom of a duodenal ulcer.
     E **True**   Although the mortality rate is low below the age of
                    60 years, it is about 10 per cent in the majority of
                    patients who are above this age.

203 Adult pyloric stenosis
A   is often the result of benign gastric ulceration
B   is always marked by vomiting
C   frequently results in metabolic acidosis
D   can often be successfully treated medically
E   usually demands surgical treatment

204 The post-gastrectomy syndrome may result in
A   megaloblastic anaemia
B   steatorrhoea
C   iron deficiency anaemia
D   osteoporosis
E   renal calculi

205 The incidence of Crohn's disease is
A   distributed evenly throughout the world's population
B   similar in the two sexes
C   highest amongst young adults
D   increased in the close relatives of patients with the disease
E   now diminishing

203 A **False** The commonest cause is duodenal ulceration, although gastric cancers close to the pylorus account for a significant number. Benign gastric ulceration is an uncommon cause.

B **True** In the early stages, when the stomach muscle has tone, the vomiting is violently projectile and of large volume, and contains recognisable undigested food.

C **False** The loss of acid and chloride ions often produces a metabolic hypochloraemic alkalosis with hypokalaemia; this requires correction with intravenous saline with added potassium.

D **True** Gastric lavage and H_2 antagonists will sometimes result in decreasing the oedema around the pylorus facilitating ulcer healing. This may relieve a benign obstruction, but medical management is usually unsuccessful.

E **True** Surgical treatment of the obstruction and underlying cause is usually required. Endoscopy is necessary at the outset to exclude malignant pyloric obstruction.

204 A **True** Megaloblastic anaemia results either from the loss of intrinsic factor following excision of the parietal cells or vitamin B_{12} deficiency caused by bacterial growth in the blind duodenal loop.

B **True** This probably results from rapid gastric emptying or the food bypassing the duodenum and failing to mix with the bile salts in those patients with a gastrojejunal anastomosis.

C **True** Iron deficiency is mainly the result of hypochlorhydria and diminished iron absorption.

D **True** This occurs in about 5 per cent of patients, 10 years after partial gastrectomy, because of malabsorption of vitamin D and calcium, it is frequently preceded by hypocalcaemia.

E **False** The incidence of renal calculi is not increased.

205 A **False** It is almost unknown in the tropics. Its incidence is highest in the northern latitudes.

B **True** This is apparent at all ages.

C **True** The mean age of onset is 25 years, but no age is exempt.

D **True** Between 2 and 6 per cent of cases have been found in the family of patients with the disease.

E **False** The incidence appears to be increasing in northern Europe. There is an association with cigarette smoking but the explanation for this is unknown.

206 Crohn's disease
   A   is confined to the small and large bowel
   B   has an infective aetiology
   C   is limited to the bowel mucosa
   D   does not produce mucosal ulceration
   E   is characterised by the absence of fibrous tissue in the
        affected inflamed bowel

207 Patients with Crohn's disease often present with
   A   colicky abdominal pain
   B   constipation
   C   nutritional deficiencies
   D   rectal bleeding
   E   tender abdominal masses

206 A **False**   It may occur throughout the gastrointestinal tract
from mouth to anus and may rarely involve the
female genital tract.
B **False**   Repeated attempts to identify any infective agent
have so far failed.
C **False**   Lymphoedema is almost always present in the
affected bowel and mesentery – this is associated
with a granulomatous inflammatory process
spreading through the whole thickness of the bowel
wall.
D **False**   The mucosal surface becomes oedematous and
interrupted by longitudinal ulcers producing the
typical 'cobblestone' appearance.
E **False**   There is always extensive fibrosis associated with the
inflammatory process. This results in the frequent
development of stenotic bowel lesions.

207 A **True**   This is the commonest symptom and is related to the
increased motility proximal to a partially obstructed
bowel.
B **False**   Diarrhoea is almost always present, being the result
of partial obstruction, impaired absorption of fluid
and bile salts by the diseased bowel, bacterial
proliferation in a stagnant loop or any combination of
these factors.
C **True**   Bacterial proliferation in stagnant loops of small
bowel impairs food absorption, leads to multiple
vitamin deficiencies, macrocytic anaemia and
steatorrhoea. Loss of weight also results from the
anorexia which marks the acute disease.
D **True**   Occult blood loss is almost always present: patients
with colonic or rectal Crohn's may well present with
rectal bleeding.
E **True**   Transmural inflammation of the bowel often leads to
fistulation and localised abscesses around the bowel.

208 Systemic manifestations of Crohn's disease include
    A   arthralgia
    B   finger clubbing
    C   growth retardation
    D   alopecia
    E   pyoderma gangrenosum

209 In the treatment of patients with Crohn's disease
    A   medical methods have no part to play
    B   surgery should be the primary method of treatment
    C   surgical excision of affected bowel is recommended
    D   steroids may provide a remission in the progress of the
        disease
    E   a high bulk diet should be considered

208 A **True**   Arthralgia and arthritis are commonly associated, particularly in the young patient with Crohn's.
    B **True**   Finger clubbing will be found in up to 40 per cent of adults with the disease. It regresses when the disease becomes quiescent.
    C **True**   Growth retardation is frequently associated with childhood Crohn's and is associated too with delayed sexual maturation in the presence of normal endocrinological parameters. It is due to malnutrition resulting from reduced food intake, intestinal blood and protein loss and malabsorption.
    D **False** There is no recognised association.
    E **True**   There is a rare but well-proven association between this condition and Crohn's disease – the reason for which is at present unknown.

209 A **False** Though no drug at present is known to permanently alter the course of the disease, a great improvement can be achieved by supportive measures, e.g. codeine and diphenoxylate will improve the diarrhoea and abdominal cramps; cholestyramine may reduce the faecal water loss by binding bile salts; steatorrhoea may be improved by a low fat diet and antibiotics which deal with the bacteria of a stagnant loop; iron, vitamin B_{12} and folate may be required to deal with anaemia and the use of an elemental diet or parenteral hyperalimentation may improve the patient's nutrition. Salazopyrin is widely used to reduce the frequency of recurrence.
    B **False** Though surgery has a large part to play, it is only indicated to deal with the complications such as intestinal obstruction, inflammatory masses or abscesses in the abdomen, internal or external bowel fistulae and indolent anal lesions. Surgery should not be undertaken in the absence of these complications.
    C **False** Since it is a multifocal disease, resection of any part of the bowel is not helpful except if there is an abscess, stricture or fistula.
    D **True**   Steroids will induce a remission in the majority of patients and thus have a role in management of the acute case. Prolonged use, however, does not confer further benefit to the patient.
    E **False** This is likely to accentuate those symptoms produced by stenotic bowel lesions.

210 Tumours of the small bowel
A are rare
B may be an inherited disorder
C most commonly present with overt or occult rectal bleeding
D most commonly present in childhood
E most commonly arise in the duodenum

211 Carcinoid tumours of the gastrointestinal tract
A are most commonly located in the appendix
B are usually malignant
C arise in the submucosa
D are frequently the cause of gastrointestinal haemorrhage
E are usually multiple

212 The carcinoid syndrome
A characteristically includes abdominal cramps
B is produced by the release of vasoconstricting substances from the tumour
C occurs most commonly with metastatic carcinoid tumours
D is usually cured by excision of the primary tumour
E can be treated successfully by prostaglandin inhibitors

210 A **True**   They only account for 1 to 2 per cent of all
gastrointestinal tumours.
    B **True**   Intestinal polyposis with melanin pigmentation of the
lips, oral mucosa, and palmar and plantar skin is
inherited as a Mendelian dominant (Peutz–Jeghers
syndrome).
    C **False** Intestinal obstruction is more common. This is
caused by an intussusception or by the annular
intramural spread of a malignant tumour.
    D **False** The majority of patients present after the age of 45
years.
    E **True**   More than 25 per cent of all small bowel neoplasms
arise in the duodenum.

211 A **True**   Whilst they are found throughout the gastrointestinal
tract, the appendix is the commonest site, followed
by the small intestine. Bronchial, ovarian and bladder
carcinoids also occur.
    B **False** The majority are benign, particularly those of the
appendix. About 30 per cent of small bowel
carcinoids do metastasise.
    C **True**   They arise from granular cells in the crypts of
Lieberkühn and grow in the submucosa.
    D **False** Mucosal ulceration is uncommon, thus bleeding is
rare. A more common complication is intestinal
obstruction. Appendiceal carcinoids may initiate
luminal obstruction and cause appendicitis.
    E **False** Multiplicity is very uncommon.

212 A **True**   These occur together with flushing over the upper
half of the body, diarrhoea, wheezing and dyspnoea.
The symptoms are often precipitated by food.
    B **False** Vasodilator substances, serotonin, β-hydroxy-
indoleacetic acid, kallikrein and histamine are
released by the tumour.
    C **True**   The appearance of the syndrome nearly always
indicates hepatic metastases. Although primary
carcinoids produce the vasodilator substances,
systemic effects are uncommon for they are
inactivated on their passage through the liver.
    D **False** Reduction of the tumour burden may improve but
not cure the syndrome.
    E **False** Pharmacological treatment is not yet successful.

213   Chronic radiation injury to the intestinal tract
   A   typically presents with mucosal atrophy
   B   often presents with perforation of the bowel
   C   frequently presents with intestinal obstruction
   D   may present with malabsorption
   E   is generally managed by surgical excision of the affected
       bowel

214   Acute radiation injury to the intestinal tract
   A   commonly presents with intestinal perforation
   B   produces a picture of severe gastroenteritis
   C   characteristically produces sloughing of the intestinal
       mucosa
   D   is rarely seen when the therapeutic doses of radiation are
       given to the abdomen and pelvis
   E   is not seen when the patient is exposed to less than 400 rads

215   Patients with the 'blind-loop' syndrome often
   A   present with signs of malnutrition
   B   present as a complication of Crohn's disease
   C   respond to treatment with oral penicillin
   D   show a reduced excretion of vitamin B_{12} after an
       intramuscular injection of the vitamin
   E   can be treated successfully with surgery

213 A **False** The injury produces a progressive vasculitis and an associated fibrosis. Epithelial damage, if it occurs, is probably due to the resultant tissue hypoxia.

B **True** The impaired blood supply and progressive fibrosis
C **True** result in the intestine becoming thick walled and
D **True** stenotic with loops bound to each other by fibrous adhesions. Ulceration and perforation of the bowel may occur. Partial or complete obstruction is common and malabsorption may result from the stagnation of the bowel contents.

E **False** Surgical excision has a high morbidity and mortality; bypass has rather less. In the absence of severe symptoms supportive medical care is advised.

---

214 A **False** The most vulnerable cells are those of the mucous
B **True** membranes and high does will result in sloughing of
C **True** the mucosa, haemorrhage and diarrhoea. Perforation does not occur in the acute stage but may occur later.

D **False** Nausea, vomiting, intestinal cramps and diarrhoea are common when the pelvis is irradiated for carcinoma of the cervix or when the abdomen is irradiated in the treatment of testicular tumours. These effects subside after cessation of therapy and generally require only symptomatic relief.

E **False** The effects of irradiation are related to the size of the field to which the body is exposed. 400 rads is the LD_{50} for whole body radiation injury. Whole body exposure to this and smaller doses may result in intestinal injury amongst other effects.

---

215 A **True** Anaemia, vitamin deficiencies, diarrhoea, steatorrhoea and weight loss may result from intestinal malabsorption resulting from this stagnant loop of bowel.

B **True** Any disorder which produces stagnation of bowel contents with bacterial overgrowth, such as multiple diverticula, strictures or a surgical intestinal bypass may produce the 'blind-loop' syndrome.

C **False** Broad spectrum antibiotics which control the overgrowth of Gram-negative organisms are more appropriate as a short term form of treatment.

D **True** The Schilling test reveals a lower than normal excretion of vitamin B_{12} which does not improve with the addition of intrinsic factor.

E **True** Excision of the strictured or stagnant bowel is beneficial but bypass of the affected segment will not improve either the stagnation or the malabsorption that results from it.

216 A Meckel's diverticulum of the small intestine

    A   is situated at the jejuno-ileal junction

    B   contains all coats of intestinal wall

    C   may be associated with a fibrous band connecting it to the umbilicus

    D   most commonly presents as diverticulitis

    E   is usually asymptomatic and harmless

216 A **False** It occurs in the terminal ileum between 50 and 100 cm from the ileocaecal valve in 0.5 to 4 per cent of people.
     B **True**   This is a developmental anomaly in which the vitello-
     C **True**   intestinal duct fails to close at its intestinal end. All coats of intestinal wall are present and there may also be a fibrous cord or, rarely, a fistulous tract between the umbilicus and the diverticulum.
     D **False** Bleeding due to peptic ulceration arising from heterotopic gastric tissue is the commonest complication. The next commonest is intestinal obstruction usually caused by volvulus of the gut around the fibrous band attached to the umbilicus. Diverticulitis occurs in less than 25 per cent of symptomatic cases. Excision of the diverticulum is only recommended in symptomatic cases.
     E **True**   The diverticulum rarely produces trouble.

11 Colon, rectum and anus

217 Diverticular disease of the large bowel

A is most common in the tropics
B increases in incidence with advancing age
C is associated with hypertrophied muscle in the sigmoid colon
D is precancerous
E does not affect the rectum

218 Diverticular disease of the colon

A is usually asymptomatic
B often presents with lower abdominal pain
C may present with peritonitis
D may present with severe rectal haemorrhage
E may produce urinary symptoms

217 A **False** There is a very low incidence in tropical countries.
   B **True** It is rare below 35 years and the majority of western people have colonic diverticula by the age of 65.
   C **True** In diverticular disease higher pressures than usual are developed in the sigmoid colon and this is associated with hypertrophy of the circular muscle coat. Diverticula of mucous membrane develop at sites where blood vessels pierce the muscle wall.
   D **False** Both colonic cancer and diverticular disease are common in western countries, they therefore frequently coexist. However, no causal relationship has been shown to exist between them.
   E **True** Diverticular disease rarely, if ever, affects the rectum.

218 A **True** Uncomplicated and asymptomatic diverticular disease is present in more than half of the population over 50 years of age. Less than 10 per cent of cases are symptomatic.
   B **True** Occlusion of the neck of a diverticulum leads to inflammation and oedema in the wall of the bowel which then occludes neighbouring diverticula. The sigmoid colon becomes tender and pericolic inflammation may occur with the formation of abscesses.
   C **True** Abscesses may resolve but perforation into the peritoneal cavity, or an adjacent viscus, produces peritonitis or an internal fistula.
   D **True** Occult rectal bleeding is rarely present during these attacks of inflammation but occasionally severe haemorrhage from a vessel in the base of a diverticulum produces massive rectal bleeding.
   E **True** The inflamed colon frequently lies alongside the urinary bladder and produces urinary frequency. Rarely a colovesical fistula develops which results in gross and prolonged urinary tract infections, occasionally marked by characteristic pneumaturia.

219   Uncomplicated diverticular disease of the colon
   A   can be most effectively treated with antispasmodics
   B   can be most effectively treated with a high residue diet
   C   frequently requires surgical resection of the sigmoid colon
   D   may require long term antibiotic therapy
   E   is best monitored by colonoscopy

220   In ulcerative colitis
   A   the colonic mucosa demonstrates multiple wide ulcers and inflammatory changes
   B   there is segmental fibrosis of the colonic wall
   C   colonic pseudopolyps are a feature of the early stages of the disease
   D   extensive inflammatory changes also occur in the ileum
   E   there may be associated changes in the other parts of the gastrointestinal tract

219 A **False** There is no antispasmodic agent producing proven benefit in this disease.
     B **True**   A high bulk diet, containing large amounts of unabsorbed fibre, will increase the faecal bulk, reduce the colonic pressures and halt the progression of the pathological process.
     C **False** Surgery should be reserved for the complications of diverticular disease and those cases in which the diagnosis of colonic cancer cannot be excluded.
     D **False** There is no evidence that prophylactic antibiotics will reduce the attacks of inflammation.
     E **False** Symptoms are the most appropriate aspect to observe. Colonoscopy yields no extra relevant evidence and, moreover, is frequently difficult to undertake in the narrowed, rather rigid loops of the sigmoid colon.

220 A **True**   This is the fundamental pathological change, the aetiology of which is unknown.
     B **True**   Repeated attacks of inflammation thin the mucosal surface and extend the inflammatory process into the muscularis mucosae and eventually the muscular layers of the colonic walls. Fibrosis, resulting in shortening and stricture formation, may then occur.
     C **False** Pseudopolyps are the result of repeated attacks of inflammation and ulceration and may be regarded as abnormal regeneration of colonic mucosa.
     D **False** Much attention was given to an associated mild ileitis and it was thought that this represented an extension of the colonic disease to the small bowel. It is now thought more likely that it results from backwash of abnormal colonic contents through an incompetent ileocaecal valve.
     E **False** The only gastrointestinal changes are in the colon and rectum.

221 Ulcerative colitis

    A is more common in males than females

    B appears most commonly between the ages of 20 and 30 years

    C usually presents with abdominal discomfort and diarrhoea

    D can usually be diagnosed on sigmoidoscopic examination

    E may have an infective cause

222 In patients with ulcerative colitis a barium enema examination

    A should not be performed unless the disease is quiescent

    B often demonstrates a smooth and thinned colon

    C is of value in confirming the presence of proctitis

    D is necessary for the patients' future medical or surgical management

    E is a reliable form of surveillance

221 A **False** There is an increased incidence in females (1.5:1).
B **True** Though the majority of patients present in early adult life, increasing numbers of patients are now presenting in old age.
C **True** These two symptoms together with rectal bleeding are by far the most common. Fever, joint effusions and pain, uveitis and erythema nodosum are associated symptoms in a minority of cases.
D **True** Almost all cases of ulcerative colitis have an associated proctitis, and sigmoidoscopy shows a granular oedematous mucosa which is friable and bleeds easily. Rectal biopsies will confirm the diagnosis.
E **True** Acute *Salmonella* infections usually present in a very similar manner to non-specific colitis. Stool cultures are necessary to exclude infective causes of any acute colitis.

222 A **False** Though it is dangerous to perform this examination in patients suffering from acute and severe forms of the disease it can be performed safely at other times.
B **True** Lack of haustration and a decreased colonic calibre
C **False** indicate chronic colitis. It is usually difficult to estimate the extent of mucosal ulceration and inflammation particularly of the rectum.
D **True** The demonstration of chronic colitis with stenotic areas or suspected carcinoma is helpful when considering future management.
E **False** The patient with total chronic colitis requires surveillance of the whole colon every 2 to 3 years. This is more accurately achieved by colonoscopy.

223 Surgical treatment of ulcerative colitis
   A   is usually by subtotal collectomy
   B   is usually undertaken as an urgent measure
   C   may reduce the risk of colonic cancer
   D   is often indicated for colitis confined to the rectosigmoid
       region
   E   is usually a desirable alternative to long term medical
       treatment

224 Long term medical management of total ulcerative colitis
   A   is usually indicated in patients with total colonic involvement
   B   is usually indicated in children
   C   is effective in the majority of patients
   D   includes intravenous pitressin in acute exacerbations
   E   frequently is curative

223 A **False** Total proctocolectomy is the most usual choice of operation, though a case can be made out for rectal preservation if it is not severely affected. In such cases careful observation of the rectal stump is obligatory to avoid the risk of cancer developing.

B **False** Elective surgery is the general rule. Toxic dilatation of the colon, acute perforation and severe haemorrhage necessitate emergency surgery but fortunately these complications are rare.

C **True** In total colitis there is a cumulative risk of colonic cancer developing – initially the risk is low but after 20 years of the disease it rises at 5 per cent per annum. After 25 years there is a 40 per cent risk of developing cancer, thus prophylactic colectomy is being more frequently undertaken in long-standing cases.

D **False** Less than 5 per cent of these cases require colonic operations. There is no increased risk of malignant change developing in this form of the disease.

E **False** Surgery is only required for acute complications, the cachexia of severe unrelenting disease, as a prophylactic against cancer developing or suspected or actual cancer. These cases form the minority.

224 A **False**
B **False**
C **True**
D **False**
Children, the aged, patients with total colonic involvement and those patients with severe attacks are all in a 'high risk' category wherein relapses are frequent. Medical management is generally unsatisfactory in these groups of patients. The remainder can be managed medically with symptomatic measures such as sedatives, anti-diarrhoeal drugs, vitamins and iron. Sulphasalazine, and its derivatives, should be used as maintenance therapy. It has been shown to reduce the incidence of relapse. Steroid enemata are of use in the acute attack and these may be supplemented by systemic steroids or ACTH for a short time.

E **False** Total colitis of the non-infective type rarely if ever resolves completely.

225 Crohn's disease of the rectum
  A is associated with an anal fissure or fistula in the majority of cases
  B may produce a diffuse granular proctitis
  C is usually associated with ileal or colonic Crohn's disease
  D is characterised by long periods of remission
  E is best treated conservatively

226 Ischaemic colitis
  A often presents with diarrhoea
  B often presents with rectal bleeding
  C is commonly situated around the splenic flexure
  D is often effectively managed by non-surgical means
  E may be associated with abdominal aneurysms

225 A **True** Three-quarters of these patients have one of these lesions.
  B **True** But the granulomatous infiltration of the submucosa more frequently causes patchy mucosal nodularity and ulceration.
  C **True** Isolated rectal involvement is rarely encountered.
  D **False** The disease is progressive, in contrast to nonspecific proctitis.
  E **True** Surgical treatment of stricture, fissure or fistula is not usually successful and worsens the complaint. Perianal abscesses require drainage. If medical treatment fails then severe cases will require excision of the rectum.

226 A **False** Diarrhoea is not an early feature. The ischaemic
  B **True** mucosa becomes oedematous and ulcerates. This produces significant blood loss into the bowel lumen and lower abdominal pain. The pathogenesis is frequently obscure for often no occlusion can be found in the appropriate colonic vessels.
  C **True** Though all parts of the colon may be affected the splenic flexure is the area most commonly involved.
  D **True** Many patients may be managed by close observation, blood and fluid replacement and antibiotic therapy. A barium enema will demonstrate localised oedema of the bowel wall in the early stages. Late ischaemic strictures may develop and require surgical relief.
  E **True** It is usually caused by atherosclerotic occlusion or superimposed thrombosis or embolism of the inferior mesenteric artery.

227   Acute volvulus of the sigmoid colon
    A   most frequently occurs in eastern Europe and Africa
    B   is relatively common amongst athletes
    C   usually produces abdominal distension which is most
        marked on the left side
    D   may be effectively treated without resorting to laparotomy
    E   can be readily diagnosed by abdominal radiographs

228   Hirschsprung's disease
    A   is the result of acquired aganglionosis of the large bowel
    B   is associated with small bowel dysmotility
    C   usually becomes evident in early adult life
    D   can usually be diagnosed on a barium enema
    E   can usually be managed by dietary means

227 A **True**   There is a high incidence in the western world
amongst institutionalised patients, but the highest
rates are reported from eastern Europe and Africa
where high bulk diets have been blamed for
producing colonic distension. Only 15 per cent of
cases involve the caecum. Most of the remainder
occur in the sigmoid colon where a redundant loop
usually rotates on the sigmoid mesocolon.

    B **False**   There is no relationship.

    C **True**   The patient presents with colicky lower abdominal
pain, vomiting and gross asymmetrical distension of
the abdomen. In sigmoid volvulus this is maximal on
the left side.

    D **True**   Unless there are signs of colonic strangulation the
patient should be placed in the knee-elbow position
(this may itself untwist the loop) and
sigmoidoscoped, after which a flatus tube is gently
introduced into the twisted loop to decompress.
Failure to achieve this satisfying result indicates that
surgical reduction or resection is required.

    E **True**   Gross asymmetric colonic distension with fluid levels
at different heights is usually seen.

228 A **False**   This is a congenital condition in which aganglionosis
of the rectum and part of the colon results in lack of
peristaltic activity and some degree of large bowel
obstruction.

    B **False**   There is no disorder of the remaining gastrointestinal
tract.

    C **False**   Most patients with this complaint have some degree
of constipation in the neonatal period. Only a few
cases will present in later life.

    D **True**   The barium enema reveals dilatation of the normal
colon proximal to the aganglionic segment which is
of normal diameter. Diagnosis can be confirmed by a
rectal biopsy which reveals the abscence of a
myenteric nerve plexus.

    E **False**   Resection or bypass of the aganglionic segment must
be performed. This is frequently preceded by a
colostomy.

229 Colonic polyps
A are associated with colonic cancer T
B may be hereditary T
C should not be removed if they are asymptomatic T
D are usually hyperplastic T
E become more frequent in later life

230 Villous papillomata of the large bowel
A are usually sessile
B are more common on the right side of the colon
C may cause renal failure
D rarely become malignant
E can be treated by local, rather than radical, colonic excision

229   A   **True**   In 10 per cent of resected colonic cancers there are
                      neighbouring benign polyps. There is good
                      epidemiological evidence to support the view that
                      adenomatous polyps are precancerous.
      B   **True**   Familial polyposis is inherited as a Mendelian
                      dominant. It is a premalignant condition and
                      neoplasia can only be avoided by total colectomy
                      before the age of 20.
      C   **False**   Polyps occur in 10 to 20 per cent of the adult
                      populatiorn and many are symptomless. However,
                      neoplasia will arise in a proportion of adenomatous
                      polyps; therefore those that are sessile, greater than
                      2 cm, bleeding or apparently infiltrating should be
                      removed as a prophylactic measure.
      D   **False**   Adenomatous polyps are the commonest tumours
                      but juvenile polyps and hyperplastic polyps are not
                      infrequently encountered.
      E   **True**   Adenomas, some of which are premalignant are
                      much more common in the middle-aged and elderly.

230   A   **True**   These are velvety soft polypoid tumours which
                      frequently spread to surround the bowel lumen.
                      Areas of malignant change can be recognised by
                      surface ulceration or areas of induration.
      B   **False**   90 per cent of the tumours occur in the rectum and
                      distal half of the sigmoid colon.
      C   **True**   Occasionally the loss of mucus from these tumours is
                      so excessive (amounting to 3 litres or more per day)
                      that hypokalaemia, hyponatraemia, dehydration and
                      renal failure occur.
      D   **False**   Whilst the majority of these tumours are benign, they
                      have a very high malignant potential. Invasive
                      carcinoma has been reported in up to 40 per cent of
                      these lesions.
      E   **True**   Provided that the papilloma is benign and
                      demonstrates no signs of malignant change local
                      excision or limited colectomy is curative.

231   A right-sided colonic cancer frequently presents with
   A   anaemia
   B   rectal bleeding
   C   intestinal obstruction
   D   an abdominal mass
   E   weight loss

232   A left-sided colonic cancer frequently presents with
   A   anaemia
   B   rectal bleeding
   C   intestinal obstruction
   D   abdominal pain
   E   an abdomInal mass

233   Curative cancer surgery of the colon necessitates
   A   total excision of all neoplastic tissue
   B   excision of all neighbouring related lymph nodes in
       continuity
   C   early control of the arterial supply to the tumour to prevent
       blood-borne metastases during manipulation
   D   a routine 'second look' laparotomy to detect and treat early
       recurrence
   E   regular biennial surveillance of the remaining colon by
       colonoscopy or barium enema

231 A **True** The general pattern of symptomatology of right-sided colonic cancers is determined by (i) their relatively long distance from the anus, and (ii) the fluid bowel contents of the right side of the colon.

   B **False** Bleeding does occur from these cancers but it is well mixed with the stool, frequently passing unnoticed by the patient until anaemia is present.

   C **False** Because the bowel contents of the right colon are
   D **True** fluid, intestinal obstruction is rare and the tumour frequently enlarges to become palpable or indeed visible on abdominal examination.

   E **True** By this time, systemic effects may be present to cause weight loss, particularly if the tumour has spread to the liver.

232 A **False** The left side of the colon is narrower than the right,
   B **True** nearer to the anus and its contents are more soild, thus rectal bleeding is usually overt and noticed by the patient. Anaemia is a less common presentation in left-sided lesions.

   C **True** The tumour frequently causes a degree of
   D **True** obstruction which produces lower abdominal pain and pencil-like stools or frank obstruction. Thus the presentation of patients with left-sided cancers is frequently earlier than patients with right-sided cancers.

   E **False** It is uncommon for a left-sided tumour to produce an abdominal mass before bleeding or obstructive symptoms have presented.

233 A **True** In order to remove the likeliest foci of spread of
   B **True** malignant cells.
   C **False** In order to diminish the potential risk of tumour cell embolisation the veins draining the region of the growth are ligated before mobilisation of the malignancy begins. Arterial ligation can have no such benefit.

   D **False** This procedure, though it possesses theoretical advantages, is not yet widely used. It remains to be demonstrated whether any improvement in survival is sufficient to outweigh the morbidity and mortality of the second procedure.

   E **True** 'Second' metachronous tumours in the colon are not uncommon so continuing surveillance of the remaining colon is recommended.

234   Surgical excision of a colonic cancer

  A   is the only mode of cure
  B   may be inferior in terms of cure rate to radiotherapy
  C   should not be attempted in the presence of widespread metastases
  D   should be preceded by preoperative investigation for liver or disseminated metastases
  E   is complicated by anastomotic recurrences

235   The survival of surgically treated patients with large bowel cancer depends on

  A   the absence of lymph node metastasis
  B   the degree of differentiation of the cancer
  C   whether the primary is right or left sided
  D   the involvement of other organs
  E   the use of adjuvant chemotherapy

234 A **True**   It succeeds in curing 70 per cent of cases where the tumour is confined to the bowel wall and 30 per cent of those where lymph node metastases are noted.

   B **False**   Radiotherapy is used in some centres as an adjunct to surgery for rectal cancer but the adenocarcinoma is relatively insensitive to radiation. It is not possible to safely give curative doses of radiation to the colon.

   C **False**   Removal of an obstructing, bleeding, painful lesion is in most cases the most effective palliation for incurable cancer of the colon.

   D **False**   Investigation of the patient, searching for metastases, is not routinely employed. If the primary tumour is symptomatic, some relief can be gained by surgical excision.

   E **True**   Intraluminal scatter of neoplastic cells is increased during surgical manipulation of the bowel, which may be the cause of some anastomotic recurrences. It is likely, however, that the majority of these are due to residual tumour in the surgical field.

235 A **True**   The status of the lymph nodes is a most important determinant of survival, for, when cancer is present in the nodes, the survival rate drops to half that of a comparable tumour without nodes.

   B **True**   Anaplastic tumours have the worst prognosis and the prognosis worsens if the tumour has spread through the bowel wall, particularly if it spreads extraserosally to involve other organs.

   C **True**
   D **True**   There appears to be an improved survival in comparable right-sided tumours – possibly due to the relative ease with which radical resection can be performed.

   E **False**   The use of adjuvant chemotherapy has not yet been consistently shown to be associated with improved survival after resection of colonic cancer.

236 The early diagnosis of rectal cancer may be achieved by
- A rectal and sigmoidoscopic examination
- B barium enema examination
- C faecal occult blood estimations
- D detailed investigation of all patients with iron deficiency anaemia
- E the investigation of first degree relatives

237 Rectal cancer
- A is usually of squamous cell origin
- B usually metastasises by lymphatic spread
- C frequently presents with faecal impaction
- D often causes intestinal obstruction
- E frequently requires a barium enema for accurate diagnosis

238 Rectal bleeding
- A which is bright red and occurring on defaecation is usually arising from the anal canal
- B which is dark and mixed with the stool is arising from the rectum or above
- C may frequently arise from the right colon
- D should be investigated by a sigmoidoscopic examination in all cases
- E should be investigated by a barium enema examination in all cases

236   A   **True**   50 per cent of all large bowel tumours lie within reach of the sigmoidoscope and half of these are palpable by the examining finger.

B   **False**   The capacious rectum does not readily yield its secrets to the radiologist – a sigmoidoscopy is essential before this investigation.

C   **True**   Although benign causes of faecal blood loss are very common, screening of patients for occult gastrointestinal blood loss is effective in diagnosing colorectal cancer at an early stage.

D   **True**   This will include investigation of the whole gastrointestinal tract, including sigmoidoscopy and possibly a barium enema examination.

E   **False**   Although there is a slight familial tendency, it is so slight as to render this strategy ineffective.

237   A   **False**   The vast majority are adenocarcinomata.

B   **True**   Lymphatic spread to pararectal and inferior mesenteric nodes is common. Venous spread also occurs and results in liver metastases.

C   **False**   Faecal impaction and obstruction are very rare

D   **False**   symptoms with this condition. It usually presents with rectal bleeding, the passage of slime rectally or a sensation of constant rectal fullness, and incomplete defaecation (tenesmus).

E   **False**   Many of the neoplasms can be palpated by digital examination. Barium enema examinations will demonstrate associated colonic pathology but are imprecise in the examination of the rectum.

238   A   **True**   In these cases the blood is not mixed with the stool.

B   **True**   Decomposition of the blood and some mixing with the stool occurs when bleeding is from the rectum or above.

C   **False**   Caecal or right colonic bleeding usually produces blackening of the stools (melaena) unless it is brisk and in those circumstances cardiovascular changes will also be present.

D   **True**   If the history suggests anal canal bleeding and

E   **False**   proctosigmoidoscopy confirms this and verifies that there is no other cause in the lowest 25 cm of the gastrointestinal tract, a barium enema need not be undertaken. However, a barium enema is necessary if the sigmoidoscopy is normal.

239 Haemorrhoids
  A   are caused by varicosities in anal veins
  B   usually cause pruritus
  C   are often associated with intense pain
  D   often become infected
  E   will often resolve after conservative treatment

240 An anal fistula
  A   is usually a congenital condition
  B   often presents with pruritus
  C   may be associated with chronic colonic inflammation
  D   can be successfully treated with a low residue diet
  E   may be caused by perianal abscess

241 An anal fissure
  A   is an ulcer of the anal mucosa
  B   usually lies anteriorly
  C   is more common in men
  D   may be associated with a hypertrophied skin tag
  E   can usually, in acute cases be treated conservatively

239 A **False** They are swollen anal cushions and commonly the result of straining at stool. They become congested with blood but no varicosities develop.

   B **True** They cause prolapse and thus produce irritation of the anal skin. Some mucous discharge follows and the perianal skin becomes excoriated and pruritic.

   C **True** Uncomplicated internal haemorrhoids are usually painless. Internal haemorrhoidal thrombosis, which is uncommon, produces severe anal pain which may not be relieved until haemorrhoidectomy is performed. External haemorrhoidal thrombosis is more common and very painful for 3 to 5 days.

   D **False** This is an unusual complication.

   E **True** Attention to bowel habit by the prescription of a high fibre diet will help minor haemorrhoids to regress.

240 A **False** This is an acquired condition usually arising from infected anal glands.

   B **True** The discharging sinus results in maceration of the perianal skin and pruritus.

   C **True** 30 per cent of patients with colonic Crohn's disease also possess anal fissures or fistulae. There is a high incidence also in chronic ulcerative colitis.

   D **False** Only surgical excision of all the sinus tract will result in cure.

   E **True** Perianal abscesses are usually caused by infections of anal glands at the anorectal junction. If they discharge onto the perianal skin, or are incised, an anal fistula is the usual outcome.

241 A **True** It is a linear ulcer of the anal canal usually lying
   B **False** posteriorly. Constipation is a common cause; it
   C **False** causes intense pain during defaecation and is more common in women.

   D **True** Chronic fissures are often evident by a tag of skin, the sentinel tag.

   E **True** The majority of acute fissures will heal with a laxative and local anaesthetic cream but if this fails a firm digital stretch under anaesthesia is usually curative. It is important to remember that the condition is common in Crohn's disease, although it may be confused with a squamous cell cancer of the anal canal.

242   Perianal abscesses
    A   commence in the anal wall
    B   have the same aetiology as ischiorectal abscesses
    C   are effectively treated by antibiotics
    D   may result in a fistula-in-ano
    E   are frequent complications of ulcerative colitis

243   Rectal prolapse
    A   is commonly seen in infants
    B   is commonly seen in the elderly
    C   is often associated with poor anal tone
    D   may result from severe constipation
    E   may in some cases be successfully treated by
        haemorrhoidectomy

244   Carcinoma of the anus
    A   is generally an adenocarcinoma
    B   readily spreads to the inguinal lymph nodes
    C   has a similar prognosis to rectal carcinoma
    D   should usually be treated by an abdominoperineal resection
        of rectum
    E   may have an infective cause

242 A **True**   Both ischiorectal and perianal abscesses usually arise
     B **True**   from intersphincteric abscesses arising from infected
                   anal glands.
     C **False**   Antibiotics will not resolve established abscesses;
                   early incision and drainage is required.
     D **True**   If the infection does not completely resolve, it is likely
                   that a fistula-in-ano will result.
     E **False**   There is no association with ulcerative colitis but they
                   are common in Crohn's disease affecting the anal
                   canal.

243 A **True**   The disease commonly occurs in both age groups. It
     B **True**   is particularly common amongst elderly childless
                   women. In infants it is not a chronic condition and
                   frequently resolves without treatment.
     C **True**   This is most usual in the elderly and is associated
                   with faecal incontinence.
     D **False**   It is almost always the result of intussusception of
                   the anterior rectal wall as a consequence of poor
                   tone in the muscles of the pelvic floor.
     E **True**   For mild degrees of prolapse in the elderly, a
                   mucosal resection is sufficient treatment; other
                   patients may need some form of rectal fixation or
                   excision of the prolapsed mucosa and plication of the
                   prolapsed bowel.

244 A **False**   Squamous cell carcinoma is far more common.
     B **True**   It reaches these nodes via the lymphatics of the
                   perianal skin.
     C **True**   There is an overall 5-years survival rate of 40 per cent
                   in both neoplasms.
     D **False**   Chemotherapy and radiotherapy are the preferred
                   treatment of all but the earliest and smallest
                   tumours. In the latter, local surgical excision may be
                   employed with radiotherapy.
     E **True**   Anal intercourse appears to be a risk factor
                   suggesting that a sexually transmitted agent may be
                   important. The human papilloma virus (HPV) has
                   been found in a high proportion of these cancers.

12 The liver

245 Bile

   A is secreted by the liver following the stimulus of the ingestion of food

   B is secreted into the gastrointestinal tract following the stimulus of food ingestion

   C is secreted at the rate of 200 to 400 ml per day

   D secretion is reduced after cholecystectomy

   E contains cholecystokinin

246 Bilirubin

   A is synthesised from cholesterol

   B is conjugated in the liver

   C is excreted into the bowel where it forms urobilinogen

   D may be formed from reabsorbed urobilinogen

   E is not a component of gallstones

247 A patient with chronic liver failure frequently exhibits

   A tremors

   B disorders of consciousness

   C palmar erythema

   D a cold collapsed peripheral circulation

   E gynaecomastia

245 A **False** The liver continually secretes bile at the rate of 600 to 800ml/day.

B **True** Food intake causes gallbladder contraction and expulsion of bile into the duodenum.

C **False** Food intake has very little effect on biliary secretion.

D **False** The gallbladder performs a storage function and is non-secretory. Its removal does not affect the biliary secretion of the liver.

E **False** This intestinal hormone is released by the duodenal mucosa after the entry of food into the duodenum. It causes the gallbladder to contract and the sphincter of Oddi to relax.

246 A **False** It is formed from the breakdown of haemoglobin by cells of the reticuloendothelial system.

B **True** It is transported, bound to albumin, to the liver and there combined with glucuronic acid to form conjugated bilirubin.

C **True** Conjugated bilirubin is broken down by intestinal bacteria to form urobilinogen.

D **True** Half of the urobilinogen is reabsorbed from the intestinal tract and reconverted to bilirubin in the liver.

E **False** Bilirubin contributes to the structure of the commonest type of gallstone and is the sole component of the 'pigment' stones that complicate haemolytic disease.

247 A **True** There is a coarse tremor of voluntary muscle, in advanced liver failure.

B **True** This ranges from confusion to coma. It is exacerbated by a high protein intake or a gastrointestinal bleed because of the rise in the circulating undetoxicated protein products.

C **True** Vasomotor tone is decreased, all peripheral pulses are easily felt and the extremities are warmer and more erythematous than normal.

D **False**

E **True** This results from the liver's failure to metabolise the small production of oestrogens by the patient's adrenals.

248 The diagnosis of chronic liver disease may be helped by serum estimations of
- A alkaline phosphatase
- B creatine phosphokinase
- C glutamic pyruvic transaminase (SGPT)
- D glutamic oxaloacetic transaminase (SGOT)
- E protein

249 Liver failure
- A is the most common cause of death in patients who present with bleeding oesophageal varices
- B may be precipitated by diuretics in cirrhotic patients
- C may present with personality changes
- D can be effectively treated on a temporary basis by haemodialysis
- E commonly results from prolonged hypotension

250 The ascites of chronic liver failure may be due to
- A hypoalbuminaemia
- B increased aldosterone secretion
- C hepatic vein obstruction
- D portal vein occlusion
- E transudation from abdominal lymphatics

251 The anaemia associated with chronic liver disease may be due to
- A gastrointestinal bleeding
- B decreased red cell survival
- C hypersplenism
- D deficiency of intrinsic factor
- E decreased iron absorption

248 A **True**   This enzyme is produced by bone and excreted in the bile. Therefore both bone and hepatobiliary diseases may produce a rise in its value.
     B **False** This enzyme is increased in the serum after muscle damage.
     C **True**   Both these enzymes are widely distributed but
     D **True**   particularly highly concentrated in the liver. Acute liver damage thus produces a rise in their serum levels.
     E **True**   Albumin production is frequently diminished and the serum protein falls to 30 mmol/litre or less.

249 A **True**   The commonest cause of death is liver failure whether the varices are medically or surgically treated.
     B **True**   Disorders of fluid and electrolyte balance, particularly the hypokalaemia induced by most diuretics, may precipitate hepatic coma.
     C **True**   In the early stages alteration in mood is noted but this progresses to disorientation, stupor and finally coma. Associated with these signs are a coarse tremor, warm extremities and a mousy odour on the breath.
     D **False** All treatment is supportive and aimed at reducing the nitrogenous content of the bowel while maintaining fluid and electrolyte balance. There is no evidence that haemodialysis, exchange transfusion or liver perfusion achieves better results.
     E **False** The liver is particularly resistant to hypotension.

250 A **True**   All these factors play a part but the most important is
     B **True**   hepatic venous obstruction and the raised
     C **True**   intrahepatic pressures that follow. Ascites rarely
     D **True**   follows an isolated portal vein occlusion.
     E **True**

251 A **True**   Gastrointestinal bleeding from either oesophageal varices or duodenal ulceration is common in cirrhotics.
     B **True**   There is also a decreased red cell survival time.
     C **True**   Hypersplenism often accompanies the splenic enlargement of portal hypertension and results in a depression of all blood elements.
     D **False** This is not present.
     E **False** This is not a contributory factor.

252 Acute variceal haemorrhage
    A can be reliably diagnosed from a barium swallow
       examination
    B may arise from the stomach
    C may be treated by an oesophageal transection
    D may be treated by a portacaval shunt
    E is best treated by injection sclerotherapy

253 Portal hypertension
    A is due to extrahepatic causes in approximately 50 per cent of
       cases
    B most commonly presents in the third decade
    C which is associated with cirrhosis is due to post-sinusoidal
       obstruction
    D does not usually affect life expectancy
    E may result in haemorrhoids

252 A **False** The history of painless vomiting of large quantities of fresh blood leads to an accurate diagnosis in most cases. Although a barium swallow and meal will reveal positive evidence of varices in over 90 per cent of affected patients, oesophagogastroscopy is essential to demonstrate whether the varices are the cause of the haemorrhage.

    B **True** 10 per cent of cases will be caused by gastric varices in the fundus of the stomach.

    C **True** Transection will stop variceal bleeding for a period of
    D **True** time but bleeding tends to recur earlier than when a portacaval shunt is undertaken. The surgical mortality is similar in both procedures, being about 40 per cent.

    E **True** Effective injection of sclerosant is possible via the flexible gastroscope. Bleeding can be controlled with a much lower immediate mortality. One or two injections will cure more than 80 per cent of bleeding oesophageal varices.

253 A **False** Intrahepatic causes due to cirrhosis account for 90 per cent of cases. The major extrahepatic cause is portal vein thrombosis.

    B **False** Cirrhosis takes many years to develop and thus the majority of patients are in late middle life.

    C **True** The cirrhotic process particularly constricts the smallest tributaries of the hepatic veins.

    D **False** The 5-year survival is very poor; only 5 to 10 per cent of patients with cirrhosis and portal hypertension survive this period.

    E **False** This is a common misapprehension that haemorrhoids are caused by portal hypotension.

254 **Emergency management of bleeding oesophageal varices should include**
A frequent enemas
B infusions of hypertonic saline
C intravenous potassium
D intravenous posterior pituitary extract
E vitamin K

255 **Variceal rebleeding**
A is the major cause of death after the first bleeding episode
B is a frequent event
C can be prevented by propanolol
D is not prevented by endoscopic sclerotherapy
E may be prevented surgically

256 **A portacaval shunt**
A should, where possible, be performed in patients with oesophageal varices before bleeding occurs (prophylactically)
B carries the risk of precipitating liver failure
C prevents further haemorrhage from varices in the large majority of patients
D reduces variceal blood pressure
E can safeguard liver function in the cirrhotic patient

254 A **True**   Together with lactulose oral neomycin and
nasogastric aspiration, these will reduce the risk of
hepatic coma arising from bacterial action on the
nitrogenous bowel contents.

B **False** Fresh blood will almost certainly be required.
Cirrhotic patients have a marked increase in total
body sodium and thus saline infusions should only
be given after exceptional losses.

C **True**   Hypokalaemic alkalosis frequently accompanies
bleeding oesophageal varices.

D **True**   This produces a temporary drop in portal pressure,
sufficient in some cases to stop the bleeding.
Somatostatin has recently been found to be effective,
and has fewer side-effects.

E **True**   The possibility of vitamin lack in cirrhotic patients
should be treated with intramuscular vitamin K.

255 A **True**   Varical rebleeding is the major cause of death in
patients who have bled once from varices.

B **True**   95 per cent of patients rebleed in the first year if
prophylaxis is not attempted.

C **False** Beta blockade is not prophylactic against fatal
haemorrhage, nor are any attempts to reduce
oesophagitis.

D **False** Endoscopic sclerotherapy will, if repeated, reduce the
incidence of rebleeding by 50 per cent.

E **True**   Although total and selective portasystemic shunts
both reduce the rebleeding rate, this desirable effect
is only obtained at a cost of a significant mortality
and morbidity.

256 A **False** There is no evidence to suggest that this form of
'prophylactic' shunt surgery improves longevity.
However, once the varices have bled, successful
shunt surgery is followed by a 5-year survival of
approximately 50 per cent of patients. 'Medical'
management of this group results in almost 100 per
cent mortality over the same period.

B **True**   Liver failure is the commonest major complication

C **True**   after shunt surgery, and may result in death.

D **True**   Rebleeding however does not commonly occur, once
the variceal pressure has been reduced to normal
levels by this operation.

E **False** Diversion of the portal blood diminishes
hepatocellular function and is the cause for instance
of the hepatic encephalopathy that frequently follows
the procedure.

257 A liver abscess

  A   is commonly associated with gallstones
  B   typically produces a firm enlarged tender liver
  C   is usually accompanied by jaundice
  D   commonly produces a right-sided pleural effusion
  E   may be treated by percutaneous drainage

258 Hydatid cysts of the liver

  A   are frequently asymptomatic
  B   are common in Australia
  C   require surgical removal
  D   may produce jaundice and fever
  E   are less common than pulmonary hydatid cysts

257 A **True**   The commonest cause in Britain of a liver abscess is cholangitis associated with gallstones in the common bile duct.
      B **True**   The patient is pyrexial with pain in the right upper quadrant due to an enlarged tender liver.
      C **True**   Jaundice is almost always present and an ipsilateral pleural effusion is common.
      D **True**   Radiographs show elevation of the diaphragm, blood cultures are frequently positive and ultrasonography or liver scanning may demonstrate the lesion. Antibiotics and surgical drainage are required.
      E **True**   Ultrasonography can accurately localise most liver diseases and allow drainage by thin tubes introduced percutaneously.

258 A **True**   In its life cycle, the echinococcus has dog as its
      B **True**   primary host and sheep, cattle or man as its intermediate host. Thus the disease is commoner in rural areas. Infestation occurs by the ingested embryos passing through the portal vein to the liver where they reproduce to form multilocular cysts – many of which are asymptomatic.
      C **True**   Once the diagnosis is confirmed (by radiography,
      D **True**   liver scans, or complement fixation tests) the cyst should be removed, for rupture of the cyst may occur and cause fever, jaundice and possibly anaphylactic shock due to the dissemination of multiple daughter cysts.
      E **False** Most ecchinococcal embryos are filtered by the liver and its parenchyma. It is rare for them to enter the general circulation.

259 Liver cancer
A   is commoner in patients with cirrhosis
B   often presents with ascites
C   has an increased incidence in sheep farmers
D   produces measurable serum levels of a fetal protein
E   has been associated with the contraceptive pill

260 Liver metastases
A   commonly arise from gastrointestinal neoplasms
B   occur only by tumour embolisation of the portal vein
C   may be palliated by hepatic artery ligation or embolisation
D   are usually seminecrotic
E   can occur by direct spread from an adjacent intra-abdominal cancer

259 A **True**   About 5 per cent of all cirrhotics will develop liver cancer, and cirrhotics account for 75 per cent of all liver cancers.

B **True**   The presentation is sudden, with rapidly progressive ascites, weight loss, jaundice and pain in the right hypochondrium.

C **False**   Hydatid disease, but not liver cancer, is commoner in sheep farmers.

D **True**   All the liver function tests may be abnormal, particularly the alkaline phosphatase. Alphafetoprotein is noted in more than 50 per cent of the patients with primary liver cancer.

E **False**   Although liver adenomas occasionally occurred after use of the high oestrogen contraceptive pill, an increased incidence of liver cancer has not been noted.

---

260 A **True**   But bloodspread from lung, breast and kidney neoplasms is frequently seen.

B **False**   Portal vein emboli are a cause but they commonly result from emboli carried by the hepatic artery.

C **True**   This appears to be the case — but whilst relief of symptoms may follow there has been no demonstration of any benefit in long term survival.

D **False**   Although they appear umbilicated with soft centres they frequently have a sufficient blood supply to allow massive growth to occur.

E **False**   They occur after spread of tumour cells in the portal circulation.

13 Extrahepatic biliary system, spleen and pancreas

261 Acute cholecystitis

A is almost invariably related to the presence of gallstones
B usually presents with biliary colic
C is often associated with jaundice
D is characterised by a pyrexia in the early hours of the disease
E usually requires urgent surgery

262 Gallstones

A may cause persistent epigastric discomfort
B can occur in the presence of a normal cholecystogram or a normal ultrasound
C may be premalignant
D may be treated medically
E have their highest incidence in developing countries

261 A **True**   More than 95 per cent of the patients with acute cholecystitis have gallstones. Acute cholecystitis usually follows blockage of the cystic duct with a stone.

B **True**   The pain is felt in the right upper quadrant and often radiates to the back, becoming continuous in 2 or 3 hours. Reflex vomiting is usually present.

C **True**   A slightly raised bilirubin (about 2 to 3 mg/100 ml (30 to 45 mmol/l)) is frequently found in acute cholecystitis. Bilirubin values above this level usually indicate a stone in the common bile duct.

D **False**   Cystic duct calculus obstruction often relieves itself before the distended gallbladder becomes secondarily infected. When this does not occur cholecystitis develops and pyrexia develops after 24 to 36 hours.

E **False**   The majority of cases will improve with conservative management and though surgery may be employed within a day or two of diagnosis, it is rarely an urgent requirement.

262 A **False**   The pain is intermittent, colicky and often postprandial.

B **False**   Poor opacification, non-opacification or the presence of gallstones are always noted. Ultrasonography is the diagnostic test of choice, it is quick, non-invasive and reliable.

C **True**   Gallbladder cancer though rare always occurs in the presence of gallstones and a chronically inflamed gallbladder. This may be a justification for elective removal of gallstones in the relatively young and fit patient but is rarely so in the elderly frail patient.

D **True**   Medical dissolution of cholesterol gallstones by bile acids is occasionally possible providing they are small radiolucent and lying in a 'functioning' gallbladder. Unfortunately the treatment is rarely permanently successful.

E **False**   The highest incidence is in western Europe and north America.

263 Acute cholecystitis should usually be treated by
A   nasogastric suction and intravenous fluids
B   antibiotic therapy
C   low fat diet
D   urgent cholecystectomy
E   cholecstostomy

264 Gallstones
A   have an incidence which increases with age
B   are more frequent in females
C   usually contain a predominance of calcium carbonate
D   are formed in bile which is supersaturated with bile acids
E   may be asymptomatic

265 Cholesterol gallstones
A   are the commonest type of gallstones in the western world
B   usually occur in patients with abnormalities of bile composition
C   may form in the common bile duct
D   may undergo dissolution after protracted therapy with bile acids
E   are related to dietary factors

263 A **True**   The majority of cases will respond to conservative
     B **True**   treatment. This is followed by an elective
     C **False**   cholecystectomy, 2 or 3 months later.
     D **False**   Nevertheless, an increasing number of surgeons
                    believe urgent cholecystectomy to be desirable in
                    that it prevents recurrence of infection which is not
                    uncommon in the waiting period.
     E **False**   Cholecystostomy is only occasionally indicated when
                    acute cholecystitis does not resolve after
                    conservative management and cholecystectomy is
                    judged too hazardous.

264 A **True**   15 to 20 per cent of Western adults over the age of 40
                    have gallstones.
     B **True**   Females are much more commonly affected than
                    males, particularly in middle life.
     C **False**   The majority of stones have cholesterol as their
                    major component. It is mixed with calcium carbonate
                    and bilirubinate.
     D **False**   Gallstones tend to form in abnormal bile which is
                    supersaturated with cholesterol or with calcium
                    bilirubinate.
     E **True**   The majority of gallstones do not cause symptoms.

265 A **True**   75 per cent of 'Western' gallstones are predominantly
                    cholesterol containing.
     B **True**   The bile is saturated or supersaturated with
                    cholesterol.
     C **True**   Although 90 per cent of such stones are formed in
                    the gallbladder they can form in the biliary tree.
     D **True**   Cholesterol stones which are small radio-opaque and
                    within the gallbladder may be dissolved after 6 to 9
                    months of such therapy but re-form frequently once
                    treatment ceases.
     E **True**   Diets high in saturated fat result in a high incidence
                    of gallstones.

266 The presence of stones in the common bile duct
A   is commonly associated with a long history of dyspepsia
B   is invariably associated with jaundice
C   must be considered during every cholecystectomy
D   occasionally requires treatment by choledochoduodenostomy
E   may be treated by non-surgical methods

267 Stones in the common bile duct
A   are present in nearly 50 per cent of cases of cholecystitis
B   often give rise to jaundice, fever and biliary colic
C   are usually accompanied by progressive jaundice
D   must be considered whenever the gallbladder is palpably enlarged
E   are frequently associated with intrahepatic biliary stones

268 Oral cholecystography
A   may not opacify the gallbladder when gallstones are present
B   is frequently unsatisfactory if intestinal absorption is diminished
C   will only opacify the gallbladder when the serum bilirubin is less than 3 mg/100 ml (51 mmol/l)
D   demonstrates evidence of cholelithiasis in less than 70 per cent of affected patients
E   is the preferred method of confirming the presence of gallstones

266 A **True**   This association tends to distinguish the condition
                     from other causes of jaundice such as hepatitis and
                     neoplasia of the pancreas or bile ducts.

    B **False**   Only about 75 per cent of cases of
                     choledocholithiasis produce jaundice.

    C **True**   Especially if the common bile duct is dilated, if the
                     gallbladder contains multiple small stones or if the
                     operative cholangiogram demonstrates filling defects
                     within the common bile duct.

    D **True**   Though the simpler procedure of choledochotomy
                     and removal of stones is sufficient in the majority of
                     cases, it may be indicated if there is a stenosis of the
                     ampulla of Vater or if residual intrahepatic calculi
                     exist.

    E **True**   Endoscopic sphincterotomy of the ampulla of Vater is
                     now being employed almost routinely for this
                     condition.

267 A **False**   Approximately 10 per cent of patients with
                     cholecystitis have stones in the common bile duct.
                     These stones usually originate in the gallbladder.

    B **True**   This is a classical presentation (Charcot's triad).

    C **False**   The jaundice is typically intermittent and thus
                     distinguishable from the jaundice of a malignant
                     obstruction which is progressive.

    D **False**   The gallbladder that has produced gallstones is
                     fibrotic and non-distensible due to accompanying
                     chronic cholecystitis. Courvoisier first noted that an
                     obstructive jaundice associated with an enlarged
                     palpable gallbladder is usually due to malignancy.
                     Mucoceles and empyemata of the gallbladder
                     provide an exception to this rule.

    E **False**   Intrahepatic biliary calculi are rare in the Western
                     patient.

268 A **True**   Failure of opacification of the biliary tree and
                     gallbladder is frequently due to cystic duct
                     obstruction by a gallstone or chronic cholecystitis.

    B **True**   Lack of absorption of the oral medium, or failure

    C **True**   of the liver to concentrate it when liver function is
                     impaired, may produce this effect.

    D **False**   Although oral cholecystography is a reliable

    E **False**   contrast radiological technique of the gastrointestinal
                     tract and will produce evidence of gallbladder
                     disease in more than 90 per cent of affected patients,
                     ultrasonography is now equally reliable. Since it is
                     quicker, cheaper and non-invasive it is preferred to
                     oral cholecystography.

269 In severe jaundice diagnostic evidence of an extrahepatic obstruction of the biliary tract may be gained by
    A intravenous cholangiography
    B a barium meal
    C ultrasonography
    D endoscopic retrograde cholangiography
    E percutaneous transhepatic cholangiography

270 Internal biliary fistulae
    A most commonly arise as a consequence of cholecystitis
    B most commonly occur between the gallbladder and the duodenum
    C can result in intestinal obstruction
    D are usually accompanied by cholangitis
    E result in a subhepatic collection of bile

271 Carcinoma of the gallbladder
    A is usually a squamous cell neoplasm
    B is more common in men
    C is most common in the middle aged
    D is usually associated with gallstones
    E has a poor prognosis

269　A　**False**　If the serum bilirubin is above 68 to 85 mmol/l no visualisation of the biliary tract will be achieved.

　　B　**True**　A barium meal will yield information about the head of the pancreas and the ampullary region but this indirect and rather unreliable investigation has been replaced by one or other of the following two investigations.

　　C　**True**　Ultrasonography is the first investigation of choice; if it reveals dilated bile ducts more invasive investigations are indicated and may reveal the cause and site of the obstruction.

　　D　**True**　Retrograde cannulation of the ampulla allows cholangiography to be achieved directly and is occasionally of great diagnostic value.

　　E　**True**　Percutaneous transhepatic cholangiography may yield valuable information prior to laparotomy if the intrahepatic bile ducts are obstructed and distended.

270　A　**True**　By far the commonest cause is an inflamed gallbladder becoming adherent to a neighbouring viscus and the contained gallstones eroding into this viscus.

　　B　**True**　More than 75 per cent of these fistulae are between the gallbladder and duodenum.

　　C　**True**　Occasionally the passage of gallstones into the intestinal tract results in internal obstruction, usually in the terminal ileum, the narrowest part of the intestinal tract.

　　D　**False**　Though cholangitis may occasionally be a complication, it is rare – many such fistulae close without treatment.

　　E　**False**　The fistula is almost always a consequence of necrosis of an inflamed common bile duct wall and the bile leaks into an adjacent intestine rather than into the peritoneal cavity.

271　A　**False**　The majority are adenocarcinomas and are much
　　B　**False**　more common in females.
　　C　**False**　The incidence is highest in the elderly and more than 90 per cent of cases are associated with gallstones.

　　D　**True**　It is widely believed, but not proven, that calculous cholecystitis is an aetiological factor. The symptoms are usually similar in the two conditions.

　　E　**True**　The 5-year survival is less than 5 per cent – the tumour is usually advanced at the time of presentation.

272   Hypersplenism

- A   results in anaemia, leucopenia and thrombocytopenia
- B   only occurs in the presence of a large spleen
- C   requires surgical treatment
- D   frequently follows liver cirrhosis
- E   may be diagnosed by bone marrow biopsy

273   Acute pancreatitis

- A   is commonly associated with the presence of gallstones
- B   has a high incidence in alcoholics
- C   occurs most commonly in diabetics
- D   may have a viral origin
- E   becomes more severe with each recurring episode

274   Acute pancreatitis

- A   presents with diffuse epigastric pain
- B   produces exaggerated bowel sounds
- C   may be diagnosed by an elevated urinary diastase
- D   may be complicated by hypoxia
- E   may be complicated by renal failure

272 A **True** Hypersplenism produces trapping of the formed elements of the blood within the spleen and an abnormally high rate of destruction of red and white blood cells and platelets.

B **True** Hypersplenism is always the result of a hypertrophied spleen either by inflammatory, infiltrative or congestive processes.

C **True** Splenectomy usually reverses the above changes.

D **True** Any process which produces portal hypertension may result in hypersplenism.

E **True** Increased erythropoiesis and an excess of megakaryocytes will be noted.

273 A **True** The aetiology of this condition is unknown, but biliary reflux into the pancreatic duct and spasm of the sphincter of Oddi are thought to be important. In Britain about half the patients have coexisting gallstones. Though only a small proportion have stones found in the common bile duct there is evidence that temporary ampullary obstruction by a gallstone that is subsequently discharged into the duodenum is quite common.

B **True** There is an increased incidence in alcoholics and in the USA this is the most commonly associated condition.

C **False** It does not occur very commonly in diabetics.

D **True** As, for example, in Coxsackie infections and glandular fever.

E **False** It is usual that the first attack is the most severe. Further attacks usually decrease in severity.

274 A **True** The pain may be slow in onset but often becomes severe, constant and radiating to the back and the left flank.

B **False** Bowel sounds are diminished or absent in severe cases because of the associated paralytic ileus.

C **True** The serum amylase is very frequently raised but often for only 24 hours or so. The urinary diastase is similarly elevated but for 1 or 2 days longer.

D **True** Severe pancreatitis produces widespread systemic effects.

E **True** Circulating 'toxic broth' is noxious to many tissues, aveolar oedema results in hypoxia, sequestration of fluid often results in oliguria and renal failure.

275 Chronic pancreatitis

    A is commonly associated with alcoholism
    B is associated with diabetes
    C may be diagnosed by the analysis of pancreatic secretions
    D is best investigated by retrograde pancreatography
    E may be treated by surgical procedures which decompress the pancreatic duct

276 Pancreatic pseudocysts

    A are developmental in origin
    B usually arise in the lesser peritoneal sac
    C produce a smooth epigastric mass which moves on respiration
    D may be effectively treated by internal drainage
    E may be complicated by haemorrhage

277 The Zollinger–Ellison syndrome

    A is the result of hypergastrinaemia
    B is produced by parietal cell neoplasia
    C includes diarrhoea and malabsorption among its presenting features
    D is most effectively treated by total gastrectomy
    E requires removal of the pancreatic tumour

275 A **True**   The fundamental cause of this condition is as obscure as that of acute pancreatitis but biliary tract disease and alcoholism are again frequently associated.

   B **True**   Chronic epigastric pain radiating to the back, diabetes, steatorrhoea and weight loss combine to form the classical presentation.

   C **True**   Diagnosis may be difficult but the enzyme content of the pancreatic secretions secreted in response to hormonal or food stimulation is frequently diminished.

   D **True**   Pancreatography will reveal characteristic stricturing and dilatation of the main pancreatic duct, and in addition may allow surgical treatment to be planned.

   E **True**   Pancreatic duct obstruction is the usual cause of the progression of the disease, thus sphincteroplasty or drainage of the duct into the jejunum may be employed with moderately good results. If gallstones are present cholecystectomy should be performed.

276 A **False**   There is usually a history of preceding pancreatitis or trauma. They arise following rupture of a pancreatic duct and the subsequent leakage of pancreatic secretions into the retroperitoneal tissues.

   B **True**   They are thus commonly related to surrounding organs, the stomach, liver and colon.

   C **False**   Though a smooth mass can usually be palpated, it does not move on respiration.

   D **True**   Internal drainage of the cyst into the stomach or small bowel is the preferred treatment, provided the cyst is not infected and its wall is well formed.

   E **True**   Chronic inflammation around the pseudocyst may erode vessels and cause haemorrhage.

277 A **True**   In this syndrome excessive amounts of gastrin are
   B **False**   produced by non-beta cell islet tumours of the pancreas. 50 per cent of these tumours are malignant and metastasise to lymph nodes and the liver. The tumours are frequently multiple.

   C **True**   There is a very high acid secretion, more than 15 mEq (15 mmol)/hour. It is thought that this high acid secretion inactivates lipase to produce steatorrhoea and diarrhoea.

   D **True**   Because of the multiplicity of the tumours in the pancreas, surgical removal of single tumours is rarely successful in reducing the gastric hypersecretory state.

   E **False**   Removal of the 'target' organ by total gastrectomy is thus preferred.

278   Tumours of the Zollinger–Ellison type
A   may be associated with hyperparathyroidism
B   are more common in diabetics
C   often produce unusual duodenal ulcers
D   are frequently malignant
E   may be treated medically

279   Cancer of the pancreas
A   occurs commonly in the head of the pancreas
B   is decreasing in incidence in the Western world
C   is not related to diabetes mellitus
D   is related to cigarette smoking
E   is usually treated by radical surgery

278 A **True**   Gastrinomas and hyperparathyroidism are associated in the multiple endocrine abnormality syndrome (Type 1).
     B **False** There is no association with diabetes.
     C **True**   The commonest presentation is for the patient to demonstate recurrent duodenal ulceration after apparently adequate therapy or for peptic ulcers to appear in the second and third part of the duodenum or in the jejunum. The diagnosis is confirmed by finding high levels of serum gastrin.
     D **True**   The majority are malignant and multiple tumours are common.
     E **True**   Some authorities are now recommending that cimetidine, in larger than normal doses, will control effects of gastrinomas. Whether it can control their rate of growth and spread remains to be seen.

279 A **True**   70 per cent of the adenocarcinomas arise in the head of the pancreas.
     B **False** Its incidence has tripled in the last 40 years.
     C **False** There is an association between pancreatic cancer and diabetes. There is some evidence of an excess incidence in diabetes and, additionally, pancreatic cancer is often diagnosed within a year of diabetes appearing in an elderly patient.
     D **True**   There is an increased incidence in smokers.
     E **False** Radical surgery can only be undertaken in a small proportion of cases since the majority of patients have such advanced disease that only palliative measures are possible.

14 Genitourinary tract

280 Haematuria

A at the beginning of micturition is usually indicative of urethral pathology

B at the end of micturition is usually due to bladder neck pathology

C thoughout the urinary stream is typical of renal pathology

D in elderly males is usually related to benign prostatic hypertrophy

E is a common presentation in polycystic kidney

281 An intravenous urogram

A yields most diagnostic information when performed on a well hydrated patient

B should be preceded by a plain film of the abdomen

C first demonstrates the renal outline at 5 minutes

D normally shows incomplete filling of the ureter in any one exposure

E should provide evidence of the presence, if any, of lower urinary tract obstruction

280 A **True** This pattern of haematuria is due to a lesion situated distal to the external sphincter.

B **True** This pattern of haematuria is caused by pathology in the region of the bladder neck, tigone or posterior urethra.

C **True** Infection, neoplasia and blood dyscrasias should be considered.

D **True** This is the commonest cause of haematuria in elderly males. The bleeding arises from fragile veins over the urethral surface of the gland.

E **True** Other presentations include a mass, and uraemia.

281 A **False** Better renal concentration is achieved when the patient is slightly dehydrated.

B **True** This often shows the renal size and the majority of renal and ureteric calculi.

C **False** A normal nephrogram is present within 3 minutes.

D **True** Peristalsis of the healthy ureter ensures that it is incompletely filled by contrast. If complete filling of the ureter is demonstrated then some degree of ureteric obstruction should be suspected.

E **True** Films should be taken of the bladder after micturition. In the healthy bladder there is an insignificant residue, whereas in bladder neck obstruction there is an increased post-micturition residue.

282   Wilms' tumours
A   metastasise readily to the lungs
B   metastasise readily to the bones
C   are occasionally bilateral
D   have the worst prognosis of all childhood abdominal
   tumours
E   make up approximately 10 per cent of malignant tumours in
   childhood

283   Neuroblastomas
A   usually arise in the renal substance
B   are one of the rarest solid tumours of childhood
C   usually metastasise via the bloodstream
D   are difficult to distinguish from Wilms' tumours on clinical
   examination
E   characteristically produce 5-hydroxyindoleacetic acid which
   can be detected in the urine

284   In developmental anomalies of the genitourinary tract
A   the commonest renal abnormality is renal agenesis
B   the adult polycystic renal disease is transmitted as an
   autosomal dominant
C   pelviureteric obstruction is a rarity in children
D   the upper ureter of a duplex system enters the bladder more
   distally
E   ectopia of the bladder is due to incomplete fusion of the
   metanephros

282 A **True**   This embryonal neoplasm (nephroblastoma) usually
                   presents with an abdominal mass and haematuria.
                   Pulmonary metastases are seen in more than 25 per
                   cent of cases on presentation.
     B **False** In contradistinction to neuroblastomata and adult
                   renal cancers, bones metastases are rare.
     C **True**   Up to 6 per cent of cases have been shown to have
                   bilateral tumours.
     D **False** Aggressive 'triple therapy' with radical excision of
                   the primary tumour and associated lymph nodes,
                   postoperative radiotherapy to the primary site and
                   areas of metastasis together with postoperative
                   actinomycin D or vincristine result in high cure rates
                   (90 per cent where no metastases are present and 40
                   per cent where lymph nodes metastases have
                   occurred).
     E **True**   80 per cent occur before the age of 4 years.

283 A **False** These are malignancies of the primitive cells of the
                   sympathetic nervous system, consequently they
                   most frequently arise in the adrenals and less
                   commonly in the sympathetic chain.
     B **False** They are the commonest solid tumour of infancy.
     C **True**   This is common and spread to lungs and bones is
                   frequently seen; local lymphatic spread is also
                   usually present.
     D **False** Their nodularity and fixity, especially during
                   respiration, usually enable this distinction to be
                   made.
     E **False** Most tumours secrete detectable amounts of
                   noradrenaline precursors, e.g. vanillyl mandelic acid
                   (VMA).

284 A **False** Agenesis is uncommon. Solitary cysts are common
                   and fusion abnormalities include horseshoe kidney.
     B **True**   The juvenile form is transmitted as a recessive gene
                   and is often associated with cystic disease of other
                   organs.
     C **False** This is one of the more common causes of
                   hydronephrosis in childhood.
     D **True**   This ureter is also subject to problems of obstruction
                   and reflux.
     E **False** It is due to defective fusion of the urogenital sinus
                   and overlying skeletal system.

285 Vesicoureteric reflux

A   is mostly common due to neuropathy
B   is the commonest cause of pyelonephritis
C   is most effectively demonstrated by an intravenous urogram
D   rarely responds to antibiotic therapy alone
E   usually progresses to end stage renal failure

286 Renal artery stenosis

A   is a common cause of hypertension
B   is most commonly caused by fibromuscular hyperplasia
C   can usually be diagnosed on an intravenous pyelogram
D   should be treated by nephrectomy
E   is often associated with a renal artery aneurysm

285 A **False** Primary reflux is usually due to ureterotrigonal dysfunction.
   B **True** Making up about half of the children presenting with urinary tract infections.
   C **False** Although this investigation will demonstrate renal scarring and calyceal dilatation, reflux is effectively demonstrated by a micturating cystogram.
   D **False** More than a third of patients respond to such conservative management and the majority of the remainder to reconstructive surgery.
   E **False** This group does account for a high proportion of patients requiring dialysis and transplantation.

286 A **False** This uncommon cause of hypertension usually presents as an abrupt onset of hypertension in a middle-aged patient. (The practice of screening all hypertensive patients for the condition by intravenous urography has been unproductive.)
   B **False** The commonest cause is atheromatous narrowing of the renal artery
   C **True** A slight decrease in renal size, delay in opacification of the renal pelvis and late hyperconcentration of contrast medium (due to excessive tubular reabsorption of water) are all suggestive of the condition.
   D **False** Careful assessment of the patient's general condition including the function of the opposite kidney and the nature of the arterial occlusion lead to dilatation or surgical treatment being advised in approximately half of the younger patients. Nephrectomy is occasionally necessary.
   E **False** Aneurysms are very rare and may show as a calcified ring on plain abdominal radiographs.

287 In renal transplantation

    A a donor kidney may be used from a patient with malignancy provided there is no abdominal involvement

    B ABO compatibility between donor and recipient does not have to be considered

    C satisfactory renal function can be expected with a warm ischaemic time of up to 200 minutes

    D the characteristic signs of acute rejection include pyrexia, hypertension and leucocytosis

    E the donor kidney is usually placed in the right renal bed

288 Renal stones

    A are usually demonstrable on a plain radiograph

    B are commonly associated with urinary tract infections

    C may be associated with renal tubular acidosis

    D may be improved by a reduced oral fluid intake

    E can be effectively treated with extracorporial laser therapy

289 Ureteric calculi

    A usually present with ureteric colic

    B often result from urinary tract infection

    C frequently cause haematuria

    D are not usually radio-opaque

    E producing ureteric colic should be surgically removed

287   A   **False**   Patients with malignancy are unsuitable donors, as
               are the aged, patients with renal disease or
               hypertension. Best resuls are obtained when the
               donor organ is from a living blood relative. The most
               satisfactory cadaver donors are young patients dying
               of head injuries.
       B   **False**   Donor and recipient must be ABO compatible;
               otherwise, hyperacute rejection may occur within a
               few minutes.
       C   **False**   Maximum renal function is obtained with warm
               ischaemic times of under 30 minutes. If this time
               exceeds 100 minutes function cannot be expected
               and the kidney should not be transplanted.
       D   **True**   Acute rejection is seen during the first 3 months after
               transplantation. Some success has been achieved in
               treating such episodes with high doses of steroids
               and immunosuppressive drugs.
       E   **False**   It is usually anastomosed to the iliac vessels sited in
               an iliac fossa.

288   A   **True**   Most are compounds of calcium salts and cystine is
               also radio-opaque.
       B   **True**   Requiring active treatment to reduce renal damage.
       C   **True**   This cause of nephrocalcinosis should be considered
               when the urine pH is persistently between 6.0 and
               7.0.
       D   **False**   High fluid intake reduces stone-forming potential. For
               the treatment of calcium stones a reduction of
               sodium intake promotes calcium absorption, and
               dairy products should be avoided.
       E   **False**   But shockwave lithotripsy is effective in breaking up
               calcium stones.

289   A   **True**   This is of abrupt onset and usually severe enough to
               require opiate analgesia.
       B   **True**   Infection, statis, prolonged immobilisation and
               generalised metabolic diseases such as gout,
               hyperparathyroidism and cystinuria may cause
               urinary calculi.
       C   **True**   This may not be overt but urinalysis usually reveals
               erythrocytes in the urine.
       D   **False**   More than 90 per cent of ureteric calculi are radio-
               opaque. Uric acid calculi are not.
       E   **False**   Most stones measuring less than 4 mm in diameter
               on radiograph will pass spontaneously.

290 An adenocarcinoma of the kidney
- **A** usually occurs in the 35 to 45 age group
- **B** usually presents with a urinary infection
- **C** is often indistinguishable from a renal cyst radiologically
- **D** frequently invades and grows along the renal artery
- **E** may present with testicular enlargement

291 Tumours of the renal pelvis
- **A** usually present as a mass in the loin
- **B** are possibly due to a urinary carcinogen
- **C** resemble those of the bladder in their pathology
- **D** are best treated by a partial or total nephrectomy
- **E** commonly have a raised eosinophil count

292 Bladder cancer
- **A** may follow exposure to beta-naphthylamine
- **B** is more common in heavy smokers
- **C** is more common in females
- **D** is frequently associated with bladder schistosomiasis

290 A **False** It usually occurs between the ages of 50 to 70 years and it is rare before the age of 30 years.

B **False** Haematuria, loin pain and a mass are the usual symptoms but they may be preceded by general malaise or the symptoms of bony metastases.

C **True** The differential diagnosis from the more common condition of renal cysts usually requires further investigations such as ultrasound studies or selective renal angiography.

D **False** The renal vein is commonly involved by the tumour growing along it and sometimes reaching the inferior vena cava where it may embolise.

E **False** However, a varicocele may occur, particularly on the left side due to obstruction of the testicular vein by tumour in the left renal vein or inferior vena cava.

291 A **False** Although on rare occasions the tumour may block the ureter and give rise to hydronephrosis the usual presentation is with haematuria and clot colic.

B **True** Tumours of the renal pelvis resemble those of the bladder in that they may be due to a urinary carcinogen.

C **True** They are carcinomas arising from transitional epithelium.

D **False** Their spread is by seedlings to ureter and bladder. They are therefore treated by nephrectomy and ureterectomy, the latter being extended to include an adjacent cuff of bladder wall.

E **False** This does occur in adenocarcinoma.

292 A **True** industrial and laboratory use of this chemical is now very strictly controlled.

B **True** although a urinary carcinogen has not yet been isolated in these patients.

C **Fales** it is 3 to 4 times commoner in males and occurs mainly in the sixth and seventh decades.

D **True** schistosoma haematobium is thought to predispose to bladder cancer. There is a high incidence of bladder cancer in regions where schistosomiasis is endemic.

293 Bladder cancers
A are usually diagnosed on excretory pyelography
B are usually adenocarcinomas
C are usually ulcerating
D generally present on the bladder vault
E are usually invasive by the time of presentation

294 Benign prostatic hypertrophy
A is the result of hyperplasia of the fibromuscular capsule of the gland
B results in diminished power of urination
C results in terminal dribbling of urine
D often presents with haematuria
E rarely presents with renal failure

295 Benign prostatic hypertrophy
A can readily be assessed on rectal examination
B rarely produces an abnormality on intravenous urogram
C can be effectively treated with hormones
D is most effectively treated by surgery
E is a premalignant condition

293   A   **False**   The intravenous urogram frequently shows no
disturbance of renal function. Only large bladder
cancers will be revealed on the cystogram.
Cystoscopy is the most reliable method of diagnosis
and should be performed in all patients suspected of
the disease.

   B   **False**   These are rare. The commonest neoplasm is a
   C   **False**   transitional cell carcinoma and these usually form
sessile tumours which only occasionally ulcerate.

   D   **False**   Most lesions are on the trigone and adjacent
posterolateral wall.

   E   **False**   Most transitional carcinomas are superficial at the
time of presentation and less than 25 per cent of
recurrent tumours are invasive.

294   A   **False**   Senile prostatic hyperplasia follows proliferation of
the central periurethral glandular tissue. A lobular
growth pattern usually involves either the median
lobe beneath the bladder trigone or the lateral lobes.
The peripheral capsule of the gland is displaced and
compressed by this process.

   B   **True**   As the hyperplasia develops the prostatic urethra
narrows and elongates and a mechanical obstruction
to micturition develops. The force and size of the
stream decreases.

   C   **True**   Frequency and terminal dribbling often indicate an
increased residual urine, and dysuria resulting from
infection is common.

   D   **True**   Haematuria occurs quite commonly and results from
damage to engorged urethral veins during
micturition.

   E   **True**   The presentation is usually with the symptoms listed
in the previous parts of the question.

295   A   **False**   Rectal assessment of prostate size is not reliable for
the median lobe is impalpable. (The degree of
prostatic hypertrophy is not related to the amount of
urinary obstruction. Small glands may produce
obstruction and large glands none.)

   B   **False**   Signs of obstruction may be present and of particular
note is the post-micturition residual urine. The latter
may also be diagnosed by transrectal ultrasound.

   C   **False**   Hormonal therapy has not yet proved satisfactory.

   D   **True**   Although the general condition of the patient and the
extent of his disability must always be considered.

   E   **False**   There is no firm evidence relating benign hyperplasia
with neoplasia of the gland.

296 Acute prostatitis
- **A** is most commonly due to coliform organisms
- **B** often presents as an ache in the perineum
- **C** may be diagnosed by rectal examination
- **D** requires bladder catheterisation as part of the treatment
- **E** generally responds to antibacterial therapy

297 Carcinoma of the prostate
- **A** is an uncommon male malignancy
- **B** is commonly of squamous cell origin
- **C** usually originates in the periphery of the gland
- **D** usually presents relatively early with lower urinary tract symptoms
- **E** can be readily diagnosed on rectal examination

298 Carcinoma of the prostate
- **A** can be accurately diagnosed on needle biopsy
- **B** does not usually metastasise
- **C** usually produces an elevated serum acid phosphatase
- **D** can be effectively treated by hormones
- **E** is most effectively treated by surgery

296 A **True** *Escherichia coli* is the commonest organism isolated.
Acute gonococcal prostatitis may also occur.

   B **True** This is a common symptom together with dysuria,
urgency and frequency. Fever and rigors are often
present.

   C **True** The prostate is diffusely enlarged and very tender.

   D **False** Instrumentation of the lower urinary tract should be
avoided, unless urinary retention is present, for
bacteraemic shock may follow.

   E **True** Broad spectrum antibiotic therapy has to be
continued for a number of weeks and abscess
formation generally requires drainage.

297 A **False** It is second only to carcinoma of the lung in its
frequency.

   B **False** Adenocarcinoma is by far the most common form.

   C **True** Particularly in the posterior part of the capsule.

   D **False** Unfortunately symptoms are not present in the early
stages of prostatic cancer. Its peripheral origin
ensures that urethral involvement occurs late in the
disease.

   E **True** The advanced case demonstrates a nodular diffuse
hardness often with fixation to surrounding
structures. The early case will present as a solitary
hard nodule which must be considered carcinoma
until proved otherwise.

298 A **True** The biopsy is obtained through the transperineal or
transrectal route.

   B **False** Metastases are very common and are often blood
borne, thus the skeleton, particularly the sacrum and
lumbar spine, and the lungs are frequently involved.

   C **True** Small tumours and those with a low metabolic
activity may be associated with normal values.

   D **True** Bilateral orchidectomy or daily stilboesterol has been
frequently shown to be associated with good 10-year
survival rates, regardless of the stage of the disease.
However, in some patients the risks of oestrogen
therapy (congestive cardiac failure and cerebral and
coronary thrombosis) may be higher than the risks of
the disease.

   E **False** Less than 10 per cent of patients have cancer limited
to the gland and radical surgery should only be
offered to fit patients with a relatively long life
expectancy.

299 Urethral strictures
A   rarely cause dysuria
B   are confined to the membranous urethra
C   are frequently post-traumatic
D   produce perineal abscesses
E   may be manageable by annual dilatation

300 Hypospadias
A   is the result of failure of scrotal development
B   results in the abnormal urethra opening onto the dorsum of the penis
C   is associated with chordee
D   is associated with maldesent of the testis
E   is usually associated with bladder abnormalities

301 Cancer of the penis
A   was first described in chimney sweeps
B   is more common in the circumcised
C   commonly arises from the corona of the glans penis
D   is usually an adenocarcinoma
E   rarely metastasises

299 A **False** Difficulty in micturition is common and is often
        associated with infection of the urinary tract.
     B **False** Strictures of the external meatus may follow chronic
     C **False** balanitis; congenital strictures may occur because of
        posterior urethral valves; gonorrhea and bilharziasis
        can produce strictures anywhere along the length of
        the urethra, and post-traumatic strictures usually
        affect the bulbous or membranous parts of the
        urethra.
     D **True**   Extravasation of infected urine frequently causes
        peno-scotal abscesses and when these discharge to
        the skin urinary fistulae will follow.
     E **True**   The patient is often reminded by being given the
        follow-up date nearest their birthday each year.

300 A **False** It is the result of incomplete development of the
        anterior urethra.
     B **False** In hypospadias the urethra opens onto the ventral
        aspect of the glans or penile shaft.
     C **True**   In severe cases the fibrous remnant of the
        undeveloped urethra gives an abnormal downward
        curvature to the penis.
     D **True**   This is rare but the resulting state of the external
        genitalia may produce a state of intersex.
     E **False** This is often the case with epispadias.

301 A **False** This was so for carcinoma of the scrotum.
     B **False** It is very much commoner in the uncircumcised and
        is commonest amongst Social Class V.
     C **True**   This is much the commonest site, where it may be
        hidden by the foreskin.
     D **False** It is a squamous cell carcinoma.
     E **False** Inguinal lymph node metastases are common.
        Infection of the neoplasm may also produce enlarged
        regional nodes and care should be taken to
        distinguish infective from neoplastic lymph node
        enlargement.

302 Undescended testes

A   are associated with abnormalities of development of the mullerian duct

B   are often associated with inguinal herniae

C   usually descend at puberty

D   can usually be made to descend by the examiner with warm hands

E   should be treated by orchidopexy at puberty

303 Unilateral undescended testes are associated with

A   infertility

B   malignancy

C   torsion

D   damage by trauma

E   hypospadias

304 The spermatic cord contains the

A   inferior epigastric vein

B   deep circumflex iliac artery

C   pudendal nerve

D   subcostal nerve

E   iliolumbar vein

302 A **False** They are due to abnormalities of the gubernaculum.
     B **True**   This relatively common abnormality (which occurs in
                   2 to 4 per cent of male children) is usually associated
                   with a patent processus vaginalis and an inguinal
                   hernia.
     C **False** This is rare, and usually means that the original
                   diagnosis should have been that of a retractile testis.
     D **False** Undescended testes cannot be brought below the
                   neck of the scrotum. Those that can be encouraged
                   into the scrotum are merely retractile and not
                   pathological.
     E **False** Surgical replacement of the testis into the scrotum as
                   soon as is feasible, say by the age of 3 years, ensures
                   normal spermatogenesis and may decrease the
                   higher incidence of neoplasia that occurs in
                   abdominal testes.

303 A **False** Bilateral undescent of the testis is associated with
                   infertility.
     B **True**   The risk of malignancy is some 30 to 40 times
                   greater. Orchidopexy before the age of 5 years may
                   be effective in reducing this risk.
     C **True**   Because it is often lying loosely in a hernial sac the
                   undescended testis frequently undergoes torsion.
                   Diagnosis is delayed unless the scrotum is examined.
     D **True**   The position of the testis, often overlying the pubic
                   tubercle, increases its risk of damage by trauma.
     E **False** The abnormality in this lesion is of development of
                   the genital tubercle.

304 A **False** The spermatic cord is invested with external and
     B **False** internal spermatic fascia together with the cremaster
     C **False** muscle. It contains testicular vessels, the vas
     D **False** deferens, the ilio-inguinal nerve and sympathetic
     E **False** nerve fibres. A patent processus vaginalis is present
                   in those patients with an indirect inguinal hernia.

305 **Torsion of the spermatic cord**
   A   is associated with abnormalities of scrotal development
   B   often presents with vomiting and lower abdmonal pain
   C   often produces gangrene of the testis
   D   may initially be treated effectively by non-surgical means
   E   always requires surgical treatment

306 **Seminomas of the testis**
   A   most commonly occur before the age of 40 years
   B   are usually sensitive to radiotherapy
   C   rarely metastasise via the bloodstream
   D   generally carry a poor prognosis
   E   usually present with an acute throbbing pain in the testis

307 **A teratoma of the testis**
   A   may contain ectodermal or endodermal but not mesodermal cells
   B   has a 5-year survival of up to 80 per cent in the teratoma differentiated (TD) variety
   C   may be diagnosed by the Aschheim–Zondak pregnancy test
   D   should only be treated by radiotherapy in incurable cases
   E   is conveniently diagnosed by needle biopsy

305 A **False** The testes may lie horizontally and the body of the epididymis may be incompletely fixed to the testis.
     B **True**   Together with the sudden onset of severe testicular pain.
     C **True**   This is almost inevitable unless the torsion is corrected within 12 hours.
     D **True**   Manual correction, by rotating the testis in the direction which is the least painful, is often successful in releasing the torsion.
     E **True**   Fixation of the abnormally mobile testis (and its opposite number) is always indicated even if initial relief has been obtained by non-surgical means.

306 A **True**   Although they may occur at any age, more than 80 per cent occur before the age of 40 years.
     B **True**   The majority are radiosensitive and, since blood-
     C **True**   borne metastases are less common, surgical removal
     D **False** of the affected testis combined with radiotherapy to the iliac and para-aortic nodes produce 5-year survival rates of up to 90 per cent. Teratomas of the testis are less radiosensitive, metastasise more frequently via the bloodstream and have a much worse prognosis.
     E **False** They usually present as a painless lump.

307 A **False** These tumours arise from the totipotent cells of the rete testis and may be of any germ layer, one form being usually predominant.
     B **True**   Survival figures vary with the histological type, TD
     C **True**   having the best prognosis while the malignant
     D **False** teratoma trophoblastic, MTT, (which may have a positive pregnancy test) has an extremely poor prognosis. The introduction of routine prophylactic radiotherapy to the para-aortic nodes and combination chemotherapy with cis-platinum vinblastine and bleomycin has, with these tumours as well as the seminoma, markedly improved survival figures.
     E **False** The testis and spermatic cord are excised to the level of the deep ring. In cases of doubtful diagnosis, incision biopsy is undertaken after temporary clamping of the testicular vessels.

15 Trachea and thorax

308 **The airway of an unconscious patient**
A is protected from aspiration of vomit in the semiprone position
B is especially at risk in injuries of the face and neck
C can be effectively protected from vomit by an oropharyngeal tube
D can be effectively protected from aspiration of vomit by a cuffed tracheal tube
E should be protected by routine cricoid compression

309 **The indications for a tracheostomy include**
A sputum retention
B an inadequate tidal volume
C a flail chest
D tetanus
E acute head injuries

310 **The complications of a tracheostomy include**
A laryngeal stenosis
B erosion of the left brachiocephalic vein
C erosion of the innominate artery
D tracheo-oesophageal fistula
E persistent hypocapnia

308	A	**True**	In the 'first aid' situation the positioning of the patient head down and semiprone protects him or her from aspiration.
	B	**True**	Because of the possibility of direct trauma to the airway.
	C	**False**	Although this is a simple method of establishing an airway, it does not protect against aspiration.
	D	**True**	This is the most effective method of protecting the airway in the unconscious and severely injured patient.
	E	**False**	This is a useful but temporary manoeuvre to prevent regurgitation during intubation.

309	A	**True**	Whenever respiratory function is disturbed by
	B	**True**	sputum retention which is resistant to normal
	C	**True**	physiotherapeutic manoeuvres, or by an inadequate
	D	**True**	tidal volume (because of fatigue or insufficient stability of the chest wall), an elective tracheostomy will allow spontaneous respiration to be more effective by diminishing the dead space and allowing effective bronchial toilet. Assisted respiration will be required in patients with a flail chest and in those in whom relaxants are being used.
	E	**False**	Temporary airway control may be obtained by tracheal intubation, tracheostomy being retained for use in patients with prolonged unconsciousness.

310	A	**False**	Tracheal stenosis is usually the result of pressure necrosis and inflammation. It can be avoided by careful attention to cuff pressure and the position of the tracheostomy tube.
	B	**True**	Particularly in children when the vein may be in the root of the neck.
	C	**True**	Especially in children when a cuffed tube may erode through the thin-walled trachea into the artery.
	D	**True**	This is rare, but the likelihood of this complication increases with the time that a cuffed tube is in situ.
	E	**False**	Tachypnoea is not a feature.

311 A flail chest wall segment in an injured patient
  A   is frequently complicated by myocardial or pulmonary contusion
  B   demands that frequent blood gas analysis is undertaken
  C   does not usually require mechanical ventilation
  D   should be treated in the emergency situation by turning the patient onto the damaged side
  E   should be treated by routine skeletal fixation

312 The physical signs associated with crush injuries of the chest include
  A   pulsus paradoxus
  B   subconjunctival haemorrhage
  C   pallor of the neck and face
  D   cardiac arrhythmias
  E   surgical emphysema

313 Blunt injuries to the chest
  A   may cause aortic dissection
  B   may produce a flail segment of the chest wall
  C   may, by causing a flail chest wall segment, embarrass expiration
  D   when non-penetrating cannot produce a pneumothorax
  E   rarely involve the oesophagus

311 A **True**   Myocardial contusion may show ECG changes of a
                    traumatic myocarditis 3 to 4 days post-injury.
                    Pulmonary contusion is demonstrable radiologically
                    after 24 hours.
     B **True**   Respiration is embarrassed by a flail segment and all
     C **False** except very minor degrees of unstable chest wall
                    require respiratory support with positive pressure
                    ventilation through a cuffed tracheal tube or
                    tracheostomy. There is thus a need for frequent gas
                    analysis.
     D **True**   This stabilises the flail segment avoiding paradoxical
                    movement.
     E **False** Surgical attempts to stabilise the chest have
                    generally been superseded by the use of positive
                    pressure ventilation.

312 A **True**   This is most likely after severe crush injuries over the
                    sternum when pericardial or myocardial damage
                    results in haemorrhage into the pericardial cavity and
                    cardiac tamponade.
     B **True**   Severe crush injuries to the chest cause acute
     C **False** expulsion of blood from the thoracic cavity.
                    Cervicofacial stasis which is recognisable as a
                    swollen blotchy appearance, together with
                    ecchymoses, are then noticed in the upper trunk,
                    head and neck.
     D **True**   These are common after an injury affecting
                    mediastinal strutures. Atrial fibrillation is probably
                    the commonest.
     E **True**   Air may leak into the tissues of the mediastinum or
                    chest wall from a damaged lung or bronchus.

313 A **True**   This may be diagnosed by noting unequal pulses in
                    the upper limbs. Occasionally aortic rupture occurs
                    and should be suspected if there is radiological
                    evidence of widening of the mediastinum. It requires
                    urgent surgery with the use of cardiopulmonary
                    bypass.
     B **True**   When several ribs are fractured in two or more
                    places the stability of a segment of the chest wall is
                    impaired.
     C **False** Inspiration is hindered because paradoxical
                    movement (inwards on inspiration) of the flail
                    segment prevents the full development of a negative
                    intrathoracic pressure.
     D **False** Lacerations of the lungs or bronchi can be produced
                    by sudden deceleration or by rib fractures.
     E **True**   The oesophagus is well protected anatomically.

314 Penetrating chest injuries
- A form only a small proportion of chest injuries
- B need an immediate thoracotomy
- C need immediate sealing by any available method
- D produce mediastinal 'flap'
- E produce mediastinal shift

315 A pulmonary contusion
- A is most evident radiologically 1 to 2 days after an injury
- B does not usually resolve for 3 weeks
- C does not produce hypoxaemia
- D may require positive pressure ventilation
- E frequently presents with blood-stained copious watery sputum

316 The diagnosis of haemothorax
- A is more easily made on a supine than an erect chest radiograph
- B cannot be made radiologically until more than 400 ml blood are present
- C may require needle aspiration of the chest
- D once confirmed means that conservative measures can be adhered to
- E is usually indicative of cardiac damage

314 A **False**   Increasing civil violence makes the presentation as
        common as blunt injuries.
    B **False**   The first priority is to seal the wound by any method.
    C **True**   This is followed by resuscitation and then an
        exploratory thoracotomy.
    D **True**   On inspiration there is shift of the mediastinum
    E **True**   towards the uninjured side, which impairs lung
        function. On expiration the mediastinum moves back
        towards the injured side.

315 A **True**   The initial chest radiograph will often not show the
        extent of the contusion.
    B **False**   Resolution is complete in about 1 week.
    C **False**   Larger contusions do embarrass respiratory function
        and produce hypoexamia.
    D **True**   Mechanical respiratory support is sometimes
        required.
    E **False**   This is later followed by dyspnoea, tachypnoea and
        cyanosis.

316 A **False**   The supine film allows the blood to spread more
        thinly and it is easily missed on this view. Lateral and
        oblique views are more informative.
    B **True**   Even with oblique views quantities smaller than this
        may be missed.
    C **True**   This should be considered whenever the diagnosis is
        uncertain.
    D **False**   Blood in the pleural cavity usually leads to the
        development of an organised thombus and a
        fibrothorax. Adequate drainage (possibly by
        thoracotomy) is therefore usually necessary.
    E **False**   The chest wall is the usual site of the haemorrhage.

317   A spontaneous pneumothorax

  A   is common in females
  B   is usually the result of pulmonary tuberculosis
  C   frequently occurs in patients with pre-existing pulmonary disease
  D   is usually treated without major surgery
  E   usually requires an exploratory thoracotomy

318   In a pleural effusion

  A   500 ml of fluid may not be clinically or radiologically apparent
  B   needle biopsy of the pleura provides a diagnosis of the cause in more than 90 per cent of cases
  C   rapid withdrawal of fluid is advisable in the case of large effusions
  D   blood staining usually indicates an inflammatory pathology
  E   a protein content of less than 3 g/dl is suggestive of cardiac failure

317 A **False** The male to female ratio is approximately 10:1 and the common age incidence 15 to 35 years.

B **False** More than 80 per cent occur in non-tuberculosis

C **True** patients and of these more than half have no obvious pulmonary pathology. Emphysema, bronchitis, bronchiectasis, tuberculosis and neoplasms are the usual causes of the remainder.

D **True** Most small pneumothoraces may be treated

E **False** conservatively. Should the air leak continue to increase or embarrass pulmonary function then water-sealed intercostal catheter drainage may be required for a few days. Thoracotomy is only required for recurrent pneumothoraces and is advised in order to diagnose and repair, by resection or over-sewing the diseased area of lung, or by pleurectomy.

318 A **True** This quantity of fluid is the minimum necessary to obliterate the costophrenic angles as seen in an erect chest radiograph. Smaller amounts may occasionally be detected radiologically when loculated in an interlobar fissue or between the visceral and parietal pleura.

B **False** This diagnostic procedure is only 50 per cent successful. Thus open biopsy of the visceral and parietal walls of the cavity may be necessary.

C **False** Rapid withdrawal of large amounts of fluid (over 1500 ml) may precipitate acute unilateral pulmonary oedema. Careful clinical and radiological localisation of the fluid is necessary. Once the fluid has been located with the exploring needle, this should be carefully maintained in position throughout the procedure.

D **False** The commonest cause of a bloodstained effusion is an underlying bronchogenic carcinoma.

E **True** In neoplastic, infective and inflammatory causes, the protein content is usually higher than this.

319 In pulmonary tuberculosis
  A   the primary focus is usually in a lymph node
  B   the primary focus usually heals completely
  C   the lesion is characterised histologically by the
       Reed–Sternberg giant cell
  D   fibrosis is rare in the late stages of the disease
  E   the most effective therapy is lobar resection

320 Bronchial adenomas
  A   are usually carcinoids
  B   are usually cylindromata
  C   are liable to become malignant in 10 per cent of cases
  D   do not usually produce symptoms
  E   are characterised by hypertrophic osteodystrophy

321 Adenocarcinomas of the bronchus
  A   are equally common in the two sexes
  B   are usually sited adjacent to the hilum
  C   are closely associated with pipe smoking
  D   have often spread into the pulmonary veins by the time of
       diagnosis
  E   account for 25 per cent of bronchogenic carcinomas

319 A **False** The primary (Gohn) focus occurs in the periphery of the lung. It is often accompanied by hilar node involvement.

   B **True** In a few cases, particularly in the first few years of life, widespread bloodstream dissemination occurs to produce miliary tuberculosis.

   C **False** The tubercle consists of an area of central necrosis surrounded by epithelioid cells and multinuclear Langhans' giant cells.

   D **False** This is the characteristic finding in the late stages of the disease.

   E **False** Chemotherapy regimes provide excellent disease control and surgery is not usually required.

320 A **True** About 90 per cent are carcinoid and about 8 per cent cylindromata.

   B **False** The carcinoid tumour may give rise to the carcinoid syndrome if it metastasises to the liver.

   C **True** But bronchial adenomas are much less common than bronchogenic cancer (ratio 1 : 50).

   D **False** Haemopytsis is the usual presenting complaint but more than half the patients demonstrate bronchiectasis. Occasionally a lung abscess will result from bronchial obstruction.

   E **False** Clubbing is also absent.

321 A **False** It is twice as common in men as in women (squamous and undifferentiated carcinomas are more than 8 times commoner in males than in females).

   B **False** Three-quarters are peripherally sited.

   C **False** The close relationship of cigarette smoking with squamous and undifferentiated forms of bronchogenic carcinoma is less obvious with adenocarcinoma. There is no certain evidence linking pipe and cigar smoking with lung cancer.

   D **True** Owing to it being found most frequently in the periphery of the lung, it is often diagnosed late when both lymphatic and bloodstream spread has taken place.

   E **False** This cancer accounts for only 10 per cent of all bronchogenic cancers. The majority are divided between the squamous and undifferentiated forms.

322 In carcinoma of the bronchus
  A the overall 5-year survival is 25 per cent
  B 75 per cent of cases are inoperable when first seen
  C the mean survival of the inoperable group of patients is 6 to 8 months
  D radiotherapy is the treatment of choice in peripheral lesions of less than 2 cm
  E recurrent laryngeal nerve palsy is a sign of inoperability

323 In the diagnosis of carcinoma of the bronchus
  A sputum cytology gives 3 per cent false positive results
  B biopsy of an undifferentiated growth is often accompanied by brisk haemorrhage
  C bronchoscopy is diagnostic in 30 to 40 per cent of patients
  D mediastinoscopy permits examination of both sides of the tracheal bifurcation
  E a peripheral lesion excludes the diagnosis

322 A **False**   Although a 30 per cent 5-year survival rate may be
     B **False**   obtained after complete removal, only 25 per cent of
                    cases are operable and the overall 5-year survival is
                    in the region of 8 per cent.
     C **True**   Survival in this group is little affected by palliative
                    surgery, chemotherapy or radiotherapy, although
                    these measures may provide some symptomatic
                    relief.
     D **False**   It may be combined with surgery and may alleviate
                    the symptoms of primary or metastatic disease.
     E **True**   The tumour has spread to the region of the aortic
                    arch or the root of the neck.

323 A **False**   False positives are very rare but the diagnostic yield
                    in all but the most experienced laboratories is not
                    high. Therefore, negative results do not exclude
                    cancer.
     B **False**   The bronchial adenoma is notorious for its
                    vascularity and frequently causes troublesome
                    bleeding after biopsy.
     C **True**   This investigation allows biopsy of a lesion and the
                    taking of brushings and washings from the bronchial
                    tree. It should preferably be combined with
                    bronchography. It is also very valuable in assessing
                    the operability of the tumour.
     D **False**   Although this investigation is a most useful one in
                    assessing operability of a tumour and the extent of
                    nodal involvement in the mediastinum, the
                    examination is largely limited to the right side, by the
                    presence of the aortic arch on the left.
     E **False**   Although hilar lesions are by far the commonest
                    presentation.

324   In Pancoast's syndrome

    A   the right vocal cord is commonly paralysed
    B   collateral veins develop over the anterior chest wall
    C   nocturnal pain in the upper arm is common
    D   the growth is usually an adenocarcinoma of the lung
    E   there is wasting of the thenar muscles

325   In carcinoma of the bronchus

    A   the commonest group of symptoms are due to superadded infection
    B   the commonest non-metastatic extrapulmonary sign is pulmonary osteodystrophy
    C   antidiuretic hormone may be released by the tumour
    D   posterior lateral column degeneration is the commonest spinal cord manifestation
    E   rheumatoid arthritis is a common associated disease

324 A **False**   The syndrome is produced by involvement of the lower part of the brachial plexus and sympathetic chain by an apical lung neoplasm. Typically there is no vagal or recurrent nerve involvement.

    B **False**   Superior vena caval obstruction caused by malignant mediastinal nodes is seen frequently in carcinoma of the bronchus and is not necessarily associated with an apical lung neoplasm or the Pancoast syndrome.

    C **True**   Characteristic of this particular tumour is the development of continuous severe pain over the ulnar aspect of the upper limb, the shoulder and the jaw.

    D **False**   The commonest tumour is a squamous or an undifferentiated bronchogenic cancer.

    E **True**   The first thoracic nerve innervates the small muscles of the hand.

325 A **True**   These give rise to frequent difficulty in the differential diagnosis, particularly with viral infections which are slow to resolve.

    B **True**   Quite frequently the first sign to appear is the sudden onset of finger clubbing.

    C **True**   This results in fluid retention and a fall in the serum sodium concentration. Cushing's syndrome is, however, the most common endocrine manifestation of this tumour.

    D **True**   Cerebral and cerebellar degeneration and peripheral neuropathy also occur.

    E **False**   But connective tissue syndromes such as scleroderma and dermatomyositis do occur.

326 Malignant neoplasms of the pleura
    A   are usually of epithelial origin
    B   may be associated with finger clubbing
    C   are the commonest cause of chylothorax
    D   can frequently be cured by surgical treatment
    E   are characterised by the carcinoid syndrome

326 A **False**   The commonest primary pleural tumours are
                    mesotheliomata. These are neoplasms of connective
                    tissue origin and are believed to be related to
                    asbestos inhalation.
     B **False**   Arthralgia, fever and finger clubbing are seen in
                    association with localised relatively benign
                    mesotheliomata but not typically with malignant
                    pleural tumours.
     C **False**   Chylothorax is almost always the result of indirect
                    violence to the chest or surgical trauma. It is
                    occasionally the result of malignant infiltration of the
                    thoracic duct.
     D **False**   Long term survival of more than 2 years has not been
                    recorded in any patient with a mesothelioma. Neither
                    surgery, radiotherapy nor chemotherapy appear to
                    influence the course of the disease.
     E **False**   Carcinoid tumours make up the majority of benign
                    bronchial adenomas.

16 Lymphatic and vascular systems

327 The protein content of the lymph

A from the liver is over 5 g/100 ml (50 g/l)
B from the periphery is 2 g/100 ml (20 g/l)
C from the gastrointestinal tract is 3 to 5 g/100 ml (30 to 50 g/l)
D in the thoracic duct is 8 g/100 ml (80 g/l)
E rises distal to lymphatic obstruction

328 The lymphatic vessels

A of most tissues bear a direct numerical relation to the vascular capillaries
B of the pyloric antrum pass directly to the lymphatic duct without traversing any lymph nodes
C drain 50 per cent of the arterial capillary filtrate
D are almost totally responsible for the reabsorption of protein from the interstitial fluid
E of the lower limb have valves every 2 to 3 mm

329 The lymphatic vessels draining

A the stomach pass with the veins to the caval plexuses
B the tip of the tongue pass to the submental nodes
C the lower anal canal pass to the inguinal nodes
D the upper extremity differ from that of the lower extremity in that they follow the veins
E the testis pass to the perineal nodes

327 A **True**
   B **True**
   C **True**
   D **False** Since it is a mixture of lymph from all sources, its protein content is 3 to 5 g/100 ml (30 to 50 g/l).
   E **True** The concentration of protein in the tissues rises.

328 A **True** Exceptions being the central nervous system and the spleen which contain no lymphatic capillaries.
   B **False** This is only true of the lymph vessels from the thyroid, oesophagus, heart and adrenals, the remainder traverse at least one and sometimes as many as 10 lymph nodes.
   C **False** Total lymph production is about 120 ml/hour (about 10 per cent of the capillary filtrate).
   D **True** Only a small proportion of filtered protein diffuses back to the venous capillaries.
   E **True** These may produce a beaded appearance on lymphangiography.

329 A **False** The gastric lymph vessels accompany the arteries (the regional nodes are named after them) before passing to the coeliac and superior mesenteric pre-aortic nodes.
   B **True** The lateral aspect drains to submandibular nodes and the posterior third to retropharyngeal nodes.
   C **True** But those of the upper anal canal pass to the inferior mesenteric nodes. This is an important factor in deciding the surgical approach to neoplasms of the anal canal.
   D **False** The lymphatics of both upper and lower limbs follow the veins.
   E **False** These vessels pass to the para-aortic nodes.

330   The lymph nodes

A   of the axilla number up to 20
B   of the parotid group drain the inner ear and external auditory meatus
C   of the left supraclavicular fossa are commonly implicated in gastrointestinal malignancy
D   are responsible for the production of plasma cells
E   of the umbilicus occasionally present with metastatic disease

331   A cystic hygroma

A   is a lymphangioma
B   occurs most commonly in the second year of life
C   is usually situated in the posterior mediastinum
D   usually regresses at puberty
E   can be treated by injection of a sclerosant

332   Lymphoedema tarda

A   is a late complication of venous thrombosis
B   should be treated by varicose vein surgery
C   can be improved by postural drainage
D   should be treated with prophylactic antibiotics
E   is often precipitated by minor trauma

333   Secondary lymphoedema

A   may be caused by *Wuchereria bancrofti*
B   of the arm in post-mastectomy patients undergoes lymphosarcomatous changes in 10 per cent of patients
C   is characterised by an increased number of lymphatics
D   is characterised by dermal backflow
E   may be caused by Milroy's disease

330 A **False** As many as 30 to 60 may be present, receiving the dermal lymphatics from the trunk and arm and also the majority of the breast tissue lymphatics.

    B **True** The lymphatics draining the face also pass to this group. In malignant lesions of the face with nodal involvement a superficial parotidectomy may be necessary as the nodes are embedded in the gland.

    C **True** This was observed by Virchow who was the first to link the lymphatic system with the spread of malignant disease.

    D **True** These are involved in the production of humoral antibodies.

    E **False** There are no umbilical lymph nodes.

331 A **True** Which is usually congenital in origin.

    B **False** The majority occur in the first year. 90 per cent have occurred before the end of the second year.

    C **False** It is usually situated in the neck.

    D **False** It may grow considerably during early childhood. Regression is uncommon.

    E **True** In the neck preliminary lymphangiography is advised to ensure that the cyst does not communicate with the thoracic duct.

332 A **False** It is a primary lymphoedema of late onset.

    B **False** Venous surgery should be avoided since any lymphatics that are present follow the veins and may be damaged.

    C **True** Together with compression bandaging of the legs when the patient is ambulant.

    D **False** Antibiotic therapy in lymphoedema is necessary when there are frequently recurring attacks of cellulitis.

    E **True** This is frequently the case in primary lymphoedema.

333 A **True** The filarial larvae are transmitted by mosquitoes. The adult worm lives primarily in the lymphatic vessels and nodes, causing lymphatic obstruction.

    B **False** This rare malignancy occurs in less than 0.5 per cent of such patients.

    C **False** The number of lymphatics is not increased but they are dilated.

    D **True** This is usually revealed by contrast radiology and demonstrates stasis and distension in the skin lymphatics.

    E **False** Milroy's disease is a congenital, familial lymphoedema.

334   The treatment of acute lymphangitis in a limb should include

A   active mobilisation to allow the muscle pump to maintain lymph flow
B   incision of any associated inflamed areas
C   the use of an appropriate antibiotic
D   lymphangiography
E   venography

335   Acute arterial occlusion

A   is characterised by a dusky cyanosis of the limb
B   should be treated conservatively if the site of the occlusion is above the linguinal ligament
C   demands the urgent use of vasodilator drugs
D   of a limb is usually painless due to the anoxic damage produced in the peripheral nerves
E   may produce irreversible muscle necrosis after 6 hours

336   In chronic arterial occlusion of the lower limbs

A   claudication usually starts in the shin
B   buttock claudication is suggestive of arterial occlusion above the inguinal ligament
C   skin ulceration most commonly occurs along the medial border of the foot
D   which is severe, there may be venous 'guttering' on elevation of the legs
E   there is usually an associated peripheral neuropathy

334 A **False** Rest and elevation reduce the lymph flow and help to localise infection.

B **False** Only if an abscess is present is incision indicated.

C **True** Lymphangitis indicates a failure of localisation of the infection and thus antibiotics should be used.

D **False** This investigation has no place in the acute management of lymphangitis.

E **False**

335 A **False** A pale cold pulseless limb is typical.

B **False** Gangrene of the lower limbs frequently follows untreated saddle emboli and iliac vessel occlusion.

C **False** There are no pharmacological agents available which can improve on the vasodilatation that has already occurred in the ischaemic area.

D **False** The pain is immediate and severe and worsens as muscle necrosis develops.

E **True** The onset of this condition which soon becomes irreversible is indicated by the development of tenderness and spasm in the muscles together with muscle swelling. In such cases it may be necessary to decompress the muscular compartment by fasciotomy in addition to relieving the arterial obstruction.

336 A **False** Calf claudification is typical.

B **True** It is particularly common in internal iliac artery occlusion and therefore with severe disease of the common iliac arteries or the aorta.

C **False** The commonest sites of skin ulceration are of the toes and in the interdigital clefts. Trauma frequently results in the heel or the lateral border of the foot becoming ulcerated.

D **True** This, together with pallor on elevation and redness on dependency indicate a very inadequate arterial supply which is neither sufficient to produce venous filling nor to prevent anoxic vasodilation of the skin vessels.

E **False** This is uncommon in uncomplicated chronic arterial obstruction. It does occur in diabetic patients with arterial disease and contributes to the high incidence of foot ulceration in these patients.

337 Chronic arterial occlusion of the lower limbs results in
  A muscle atrophy
  B brittle nails
  C ischaemic nerve pain
  D paradoxical warmth in the foot
  E osteoarthritic changes of the knee

338 Abdominal aortic aneurysms
  A arise from an atheromatous vessel in approximately 50 per cent of cases
  B characteristically produce epigastric pain
  C are associated with duodenal ulceration
  D which are asymptomatic are relatively benign conditions and should not usually be resected
  E may rupture into the inferior vena cava

339 Common sites for atheromatous arterial aneurysms are
  A the femoral artery
  B the middle cerebral artery
  C the abdominal aorta
  D intrarenal
  E the ascending aorta

337 A **True**   Muscle atrophy is common and most marked when the leg vessels are occluded.

   B **True**   Absence of hair and slow growing brittle nails are common.

   C **True**   Rest pain, initially felt at night and relieved by foot dependency, is due to nerve ischaemia.

   D **False** The limb is cold and feels cold.

   E **False** The conditions may coexist.

338 A **False** Over 95 per cent of these aneurysms are atheromatous, the remainder are syphilitic, traumatic or mycotic in origin.

   B **False** The majority of aortic aneurysms are painless. However, when enlargement does occur, pain is felt in the flanks or in the back.

   C **True**   There is an unexplained increase of duodenal ulceration in patients with aortic aneurysms and rupture may occur into the duodenum.

   D **False** Every patient with an aortic aneurysm, whether asymptomatic or not, is at risk of rupture, particularly when the aneurysm is larger than 6 cm or is tender. Only in relatively small aneurysms and in very aged or unfit patients is conservative management indicated.

   E **True**   The aortocaval fistula may produce lower limb oedema and a bruit will be present.

339 A **True**   These are often bilateral and occur in association with aortic aneurysms.

   B **False** These are congenital and often produce symptoms before atheromatous changes have occurred, i.e. between 20 and 30 years of age.

   C **True**   This is the commonest site. The majority of aortic aneurysms lie below the renal vessels.

   D **False** When aneurysms occur intrarenally they are usually mycotic (i.e. infective in origin) and multiple.

   E **False** With the decline of syphilis, aneurysms at this site are now very rare.

340   A dissecting aneurysm of the aorta

  A   usually starts around the aortic arch
  B   is so-called because of the extensive mediastinal destruction
      it produces when it ruptures
  C   is associated with pregnancy
  D   is a feature of Marfan's syndrome
  E   may present with acute lower limb ischaemia

341   In the neuropathy of the diabetic foot

  A   the autonomic nervous system is usually spared
  B   the fine medullated nerve fibres are first affected
  C   motor paralysis is commonly of the small muscles of the foot
  D   the longitudinal arch of the foot is accentuated
  E   ulceration commonly occurs over the lateral border of the
      foot

342   The arterial changes in a diabetic foot

  A   are primarily a microangiopathy
  B   have an arteriosclerotic component
  C   are markedly reduced by good diabetic control
  D   are usually improved by sympathectomy
  E   can be improved by percutaneous transluminal angioplasty

340 A **True** The commonest site of origin is just proximal or
distal to the origin of the left subclavian artery.

B **False** The dissection occurs in the arterial wall and is
subintimal. When rupture occurs it is usually
retrogradely into the pericardium or distally close to
the aortic bifurcation. The effects of an extensive
dissection are due to aortic rupture or occusion of
aortic branches.

C **True** There is an increased incidence in pregnant women.

D **True** This is related to defective ground substance and
decreased strength in the connective tissue of the
arterial wall.

E **True** The dissection often blocks the aorto-iliac bifurcation.

341 A **False** Sweating is lost and a dry skin is liable to crack.

B **True** Pain, temperature and vibration being lost early on in
the disease.

C **True** The unopposed of the long flexor tendons produce
clawing of the toes.

D **True** Accentuation of the longitudinal arch produces
increased loading over the metatarsal heads.

E **False** This is usually over the metatarsal due to the
increased load.

342 A **False** Surprisingly, there is little evidence for this, in view
of the profound effects in the eye, kidney and nerves.

B **True** These are the predominant changes, occurring at a
younger age than in the rest of the population.

C **False** But good control does influence many acute
complications and the progression of the disease.

D **False** Most of these patients already have an autonomic
neuropathy.

E **True** Disease of the medium and large arteries is
amenable to dilatation and surgical procedures.

343   Thromboangitis obliterans
   A   was originally described by a Japanese ophthalmologist
   B   classically involves the branches of the aortic arch
   C   is a panarteritis
   D   is seen more frequently in young women
   E   is associated with a raised ESR

344   Raynaud's disease
   A   is caused by an abnormal sensitivity of skin vessels to cold
   B   is marked by a characteristic pallor of the hands after cold
        stimulation followed by blue and then red colour changes
   C   usually progresses to necrotic changes of the fingertips
   D   may be associated with scleroderma
   E   is permanently relieved by sympathectomy in the vast
        majority of cases

345   Scleroderma typically presents with
   A   subcutaneous calcification
   B   gout
   C   facial telangiectasia
   D   cavernous angiomata
   E   disorders of oesophageal motility

343 A **False** It was first described by Buerger in 1909.
     B **False** It characteristically involves medium size arteries of the extremities such as the anterior and posterior tibial, radial and ulnar vessels.
     C **False** Histologically, the major effects are found in the intima of the arteries and veins. It is not clear whether these are hypersensitivity phenomena or whether they are just the simple effects of thrombosis in a patient whose blood is 'hypercoagulable'.
     D **False** Thromboangitis obliterans is almost exclusively a disease in males. Cigarette smoking may have a part to play in the aetiology.
     E **False** All statements in this question are true of Takayasu's disease – a very rare arteritis.

344 A **True** The disease has an unknown aetiology and is usually seen only in temperate zones. It is most common in young women appearing in the second and third decades.
     B **True** These changes are produced by intense and abnormal vasoconstriction which follows cold exposure and then, after a period of several minutes' rewarming, an anoxic vasodilation of the skin vessels occurs. There is an initial sluggish and then a more rapid blood flow through the dilated and anoxic skin vessels.
     C **False** These changes are frequently found in collagen diseases and sometimes other diseases comprising Raynaud's syndrome.
     D **False** Collagen diseases, certain haematological disorders, occupational use of vibrating tools and sundry other unrelated diseases may be associated with Raynaud's phenomenon (see B above). Raynaud's disease, however, is the name given to the idiopathic disease defined in A.
     E **False** Less than three-quarters of the patients with Raynaud's disease are relieved by sympathectomy and of these in only half is the relief permanent.

345 A **True**
     B **False**
     C **True** Particularly seen on the inside of the lips.
     D **False**
     E **True** The CREST syndrome comprises calcinosis cutis, Raynaud's phenomenon, oesophageal motility disorders, scleroderma and telangiectasia.

346 Varicose veins
- **A** are common throughout the world
- **B** are frequently congenital
- **C** are the commonest cause of venous ulceration
- **D** are associated with an increased risk of pulmonary embolism
- **E** have a reduced number of valves

347 Commonly used sclerosants for varicose vein injection are
- **A** 3 per cent sodium tetradecyl sulphate
- **B** thrombin
- **C** ethanolamine
- **D** 5 per cent phenol in almond oil
- **E** 2 per cent formalin

348 In deep venous thrombosis of the lower limb
- **A** one of the most common sites of origin is the short saphenous vein
- **B** one of the commonest sites of origin is in the iliofemoral segment
- **C** the diagnosis can usually be made by clinical examination
- **D** tender swollen thrombosed veins are usually palpable
- **E** venography provides an accurate diagnostic measure

349 Risk factors in deep venous thrombosis include
- **A** hip surgery
- **B** aspirin therapy
- **C** malignant disease
- **D** extreme exercise
- **E** previous history of thrombosis

346 A **False** They are rare in developing countries.
  B **False** The large majority are acquired, usually in adulthood. They are commoner in multiparous women but the reasons for this are not known with certainty.
  C **False** Varicose veins alone are a very rare cause of venous ulceration. This almost always follows deep venous thrombosis and its post-phlebitic sequelae.
  D **False** Though superficial phlebitis and painful patches of thrombosis are commonly associated, these rarely extend into the deep venous system and are not normally a source of pulmonary emboli.
  E **False** Dilatation may render the valves incompetent.

347 A **True** This detergent compound is used extensively in the technique of compression sclerotherapy for varicose veins.
  B **False** This could be lethal, giving rise to systemic coagulation effects.
  C **True** It is a less powerful sclerosant than A.
  D **False** This solution is used for paravenous injection of haemorrhoids.
  E **False** This is a sterilising agent.

348 A **False** In the lower leg the soleal plexus is the usual site of origin of venous thrombosis.
  B **True** Iliofemoral thrombosis commonly follows hip or pelvic surgery and may also extend from the calf veins.
  C **False** There is almost no correlation between signs in the lower leg and the presence of deep vein thrombosis for many thrombi are non-occlusive and produce no ankle swelling or calf tenderness.
  D **False** These are the signs of superficial thrombophlebitis which is not usually related to deep vein thrombosis or associated with the risk of embolism.
  E **True** This is the golden standard against which other investigations are compared.

349 A **True** The incidence is high in all major surgery and particularly so in this procedure.
  B **False** Aspirin is widely used as an anti-platelet agent in arterial disease.
  C **True** This may be the first sign of an occult neoplasm.
  D **False** Clotting times may be increased.
  E **True** Requiring particular attention to future prophylaxis.

350 The incidence of postoperative venous thrombosis can be reduced

A by raising the foot of the operating table during surgery
B by passive calf contractions during an operation
C by the intravenous administration of 500 ml of low molecular weight dextran during operation and on the first 2 postoperative days
D by the prophylactic use of subcutaneous heparin
E by the contraceptive pill

351 Pulmonary embolism

A can be demonstrated at postmortem in 60 per cent of people over the age of 60
B can usually be diagnosed by a plain chest radiograph
C typically produce prolongation of T waves on ECG
D of the paradoxical variety has the red and white laminae of originating thrombus in the reverse of the normal order
E can be effectively treated by infusion of streptokinase through a pulmonary artery catheter

352 Venous ulcers of the lower limb

A are usually the result of long-standing varicose veins
B commonly follow deep venous thrombosis
C most commonly occur below the medial malleolus
D usually penetrate down to the deep fascia
E will usually heal when firm bandaging is applied

350 A **False** This is not of proven value.
    B **True**   This reduces venous stasis.
    C **True**   This is an effective prophylactic measure and acts by reducing blood viscosity and platelet aggregation.
    D **True**   The administration of low doses of heparin in the preoperative and early postoperative period is effective in reducing the incidence of postoperative thrombosis.
    E **False** High oestrogen levels potentiate deep venous thrombosis.

351 A **True**   This remarkably high incidence corresponds to the incidence of clinically silent episodes of lower leg thrombosis demonstrated in this age group by the I^{125} labelled fibrinogen technique.
    B **False** Changes are often absent or minimal. A lung scan is helpful and a pulmonary artery angiogram diagnostic.
    C **False** The most common abnormality is ST depression.
    D **False** A paradoxical embolus is an embolus arising from the lower limb which enters the systemic circulation through a patent foramen ovale and produces arterial occlusion.
    E **True**   This method of local administration of streptokinase has been effective in producing rapid resolution of the embolus. It has largely superseded the need to perform emergency pulmonary embolectomy.

352 A **False** Uncomplicated varicose veins even if present for many years do not usually produce ulcers, and when they do they are small and heal quickly.
    B **True**   'Venous' ulcers are nearly all postphlebitic in origin.
    C **False** The characteristic site is on the medial side of the ankle just above the malleolus.
    D **False** If this is the case, associated arterial disease should be suspected.
    E **True**   Bandaging provides continuous firm compression, preventing oedema and overcoming the increased pressure in the superficial veins of the postphlebitic limb.

17 Fractures and dislocations

353 A fracture is said to be

A closed if an overlying skin laceration has been sutured
B simple, when there is a single fracture line
C comminuted if there has been associated damage to adjacent nerves or vessels
D a fatigue fracture if it occurs through a diseased bone
E pathological if it occurs through a bony metastasis

354 In a healing fracture

A the haematoma is initially invaded by osteoblasts
B the tissue formed by the invading osteoblasts is termed osteoid
C osteoid tissue is formed in an acid pH
D calcium salts are laid down in the osteoid tissue
E the final stage of repair is the remodelling of the callus

355 Non-union is often seen in

A fractures of the fourth metatarsal
B fractures of the neck of the femur
C fractures of the condyle of the mandible
D Colles' fractures
E scaphoid fractures

353 A **False** A closed fracture does not communicate with the
exterior through a laceration or abrasion of the
overlying skin or mucous membrane. Any fracture
with an associated wound of the overlying skin or
mucosa is said to be an open or compound fracture.

B **True** If the broken ends are compressed into each other it
is then termed impacted.

C **False** Comminuted means that more than 2 fragments of
bone are present.

D **False** A fatigue fracture occurs in areas which undergo
repeated stress, an example being the 'march'
fracture of the fourth metatarsal which is usually
sustained by healthy adults after an unaccustomed
long walk.

E **True** The term includes fractures through any diseased
area of bone. Other examples include osteoporosis,
osteogenesis imperfecta and Paget's disease.

354 A **False** The haematoma is initially invaded by capillaries and
fibroblasts. Calcium salts pass into solution in the
acidic environment.

B **True** Osteoblasts invade the healing wound at 10 to 14
C **False** days, the pH progressively becoming more alkaline.
During this time the concentration of alkaline
phosphates in the wound tissues increases.

D **True** This forms callus. The amount formed is to some
extent related to the amount of stress on the fracture
site, thus a fractured femur forms proportionately
much more callus than a fractured metacarpal.

E **True** The trabecular architecture of the bone becomes re-
established and excess callus is then reabsorbed.

355 A **False** Classical sites of non-union of fractures are the
B **True** scaphoid, talus and the neck of the femur. All the
C **False** areas involved are relatively avascular. Delayed
D **False** union and non-union are more common in the aged,
E **True** in those fractures with associated infection, with
inadequate fixation and when the bony ends are
separated by excessive traction or by the
interposition of soft tissues.

356   Dislocation of the sternoclavicular joint
A   is usually caused by a fall on the outstretched hand
B   displaces the clavicle upwards and medially
C   is usually treated by internal fixation
D   very rarely causes any compression of the trachea or great vessels in the neck
E   is usually accompanied by fracture of the first rib

357   Fractures of the clavicle
A   are usually of the greenstick variety in children under the age of 10 years
B   are usually the result of direct violence
C   are frequently associated with injury to the subclavian vessels
D   can be recognised by the abnormal elevation of the distal fragment
E   are usually treated by internal fixation

358   Fractures of the neck of the scapula
A   are often due to a fall on the outstretched hand
B   are frequently associated with chest wall injury
C   are often associated with dislocation of the acromioclavicular joint
D   can usually be managed without surgical intervention
E   are often associated with fracture of the corocoid process

356 A **True**   This causes the medial end of the clavicle to rise anteriorly over the sternum.

B **True**   The weight of the arm and the pectoral muscles pull it medially while sternomastoid elevates the medial end of the clavicle.

C **True**   Reduction of both anterior and posterior dislocations can be achieved by bracing the shoulders. The attachments of the articular disc which give much of the strength to the joint will have been weakened and dislocation will re-occur unless some form of fixation is undertaken.

D **False**   Posterior dislocations may cause the medial end of the clavicle to impinge on the trachea and the great vessels in the neck. Operative reduction is then an urgent necessity.

E **False**   This is atypical.

357 A **True**   Thus displacement is minimal and treatment is usually only symptomatic.

B **False**   This fracture is usually due to falls on the outstretched palm.

C **False**   Direct trauma to the outer end usually leads to anterior buckling and injuries to the underlying subclavian vessels and brachial plexus are thus extremely uncommon.

D **False**   The proximal fragment is elevated by the sternomastoid but the distal fragment is depressed by the effect of gravity on the shoulder and arm.

E **False**   A figure-of-eight bandage provides some symptomatic relief and support. In most patients the fracture heals without internal fixation. The slight deformity presents few problems.

358 A **True**   They may also be produced by direct trauma to the shoulder.

B **False**   These are usually associated with fractures of the body of the scapula.

C **False**   These injuries are usually due to a blow or fall on the tip of the shoulder.

D **True**   Surgery may be required to reposition a fragment of the glenoid fossa. Mobility is encouraged as joint stiffness gives long term disability.

E **False**   This is usually due to avulsion by violent muscle contractions.

359   Dislocations of the shoulder joint
A   most commonly occur in middle age
B   usually occur when the arm is in the abducted position
C   usually have the head of the humerus situated behind the glenoid fossa
D   are often recurrent in the young
E   are classically reduced by the Socratic manoeuvre

360   Recurrent dislocation of the shoulder
A   is usually in the posterior position
B   is usually in young adults
C   is more common after associated damage to the glenoid labrum
D   usually requires surgical repair
E   is surgically managed by tightening the soft tissues over the inferior aspect of the joint

361   In fractures of the surgical neck of the humerus the
A   lesion is usually due to indirect violence
B   fracture line usually passes between the greater and lesser tuberosities
C   fragments are usually impacted
D   proximal fragment is usually internally rotated
E   distal fragment is usually adducted

359 A **False** They are commonest in young adults who indulge in athletic pursuits.
     B **True**   The shoulder joint is at its most unstable in this position and may dislocate with a trivial blow.
     C **False** The head of the humerus is usually displaced anteriorly.
     D **True**   Dislocation of the shoulder joint tends to produce laxity in the capsule of the joint and the joint is subsequently less stable.
     E **False** The Hippocratic manoeuvre which often achieves reduction is to pull on the arm with a foot in the axilla.

360 A **False** Like primary dislocation, the head usually lies anteriorly.
     B **True**   The incidence is markedly reduced over the age of 40 years.
     C **True**   Also tears of the rotator cuff muscles.
     D **True**   Surgery is required for effective treatment.
     E **False** The usual surgical procedure is shortening of the anterior capsular mechanism and subscapularis muscle.

361 A **True**   The most frequent cause being a fall on the outstretched hand.
     B **False** The fracture line is distal to both tuberosities.
     C **True**   Although the fracture is frequently comminuted, the bone in this region is very cancellous and impacts easily.
     D **False** The rotator cuff muscles are both internal and external rotators of the shoulder. Supinator acts on the proximal fragment producing abduction.
     E **True**   The overall displacement is not usually extensive and is accepted. Early mobilisation is encouraged.

362   In a fracture of the distal third of the shaft of the humerus

A   the distal fragment is usually posteriorly angulated by the action of biceps

B   the radial nerve is frequently damaged

C   delayed radial nerve palsy is usually due to oedema

D   late onset of radial nerve palsy is usually due to the involvement of the nerve with callus

E   ulnar nerve palsy is usually of late onset

363   A supracondylar fracture of the humerus

A   is a fracture commonly seen in young adults

B   is particularly subject to the complication of ischaemic muscle contracture

C   is held in the position of reduction by the tendon of brachioradialis

D   when properly reduced has the index finger pointing approximately to the tip of the shoulder of the same side

E   is commonly accompanied by ulnar nerve palsy

362   A   **False**   The elbow is usually held flexed, relaxing biceps, and any angulation is then anterior due to triceps contraction. In proximal fractures of the shaft of the humerus, deltoid and pectoralis major muscles both act on the proximal fragment to produce considerable angulation.

    B   **True**   The radial nerve lies close to the bone in the radial groove and can thus be easily damaged with fracture at this site.

    C   **False**   If a delayed radial nerve palsy appears, it is almost certainly due to movement and trauma from a sharp fracture surface.

    D   **True**   If this is the case, then operative treatment and neurolysis (removal of the nerve from the proximity of the healing fracture) may be necessary.

    E   **False**   The ulnar nerve is not at risk in fractures at this site.

---

363   A   **False**   This is usually a fracture of childhood; and frequently follows a fall on the outstretched hand with the elbow flexed.

    B   **True**   The brachial artery is frequently traumatised in this lesion and may be lacerated or put into spasm. When this occurs the muscles of the forearm may undergo ischaemic necrosis and contracture.

    C   **False**   The triceps muscle posteriorly and the brachialis muscle anteriorly are the closest and most powerful relations of this part of the humerus and they have a splinting effect on the reduced fracture.

    D   **True**   Reduction is keyed by traction on the distal fragment followed by flexion at the elbow. Care must be taken at all times to ensure that the radial pulse is present. It is essential to cut out a window in the plaster at the wrist so that the radial artery can be frequently checked.

    E   **False**   The ulnar nerve is not at risk in fractures at this site.

364   Fractures of the head of the radius

   A   do not occur in isolation

   B   are usually associated with dislocation of the radius

   C   may be associated with dislocation of the elbow joint

   D   may require surgical excision of the head

   E   are usually accompanied by damage to the median nerve

365   In a Monteggia fracture dislocation

   A   the dislocation of the distal radio-ulnar joint brings the ulnar styloid process anterior to the capitulum

   B   the radial fracture is usually at the junction of the middle and distal thirds

   C   internal fixation is usually required in the adult

   D   the causative injury is often a blow on the extensor surface of the forearm with the elbow flexed

   E   the commonest neurological injury is to the posterior branch of the radial nerve

366   In a Colles' fracture the distal radial fragment

   A   is dorsally angulated on the proximal radius

   B   is usually torn from the intra-articular triangular disc

   C   is deviated to the ulnar side

   D   is usually impacted

   E   commonly damages the median nerve

364 A **False** In falls on the outstretched hand the head of the radius may be damaged by impaction against the humeral capitulum.

  B **False** This is usually an avulsion injury, particularly in children before the shape of the head matches the conical form of the annular ligament.

  C **False** Posterior dislocations of the elbow joint may be without associated fractures but in other forms of dislocation, fractures are common and include the coronoid and olecranon processes of the ulnar, and occasionally the head of the radius.

  D **True** Usually for extensive comminution, to reduce the subsequent arthritic changes.

  E **False** Associated nerve injury is common.

365 A **False** The dislocation is of the head of the radius from the superior radio-ulnar joint.

  B **False** The radius is not fractured. The fracture is in the shaft of the ulna at the junction of the proximal and middle thirds.

  C **True** Though in a child the reduction is generally stable.

  D **True** Though it is probably more frequently produced by a fall on the outstretched hand.

  E **True** Spontaneous recovery usually occurs.

366 A **True** It is also dorsally displaced to produce the typical 'dinner fork' abnormality.

  B **False** The ulna styloid (to which the disc is also attached) is often avulsed but the intra-articular disc of fibrocartilage is far too strong to be torn.

  C **False** The distal radial fragment is always radially deviated.

  D **True** Therefore reduction of a Colles' fracture should include traction (to overcome impaction), flexion (to overcome dorsal angulation) and ulnar deviation (to overcome radial deviation).

  E **False** Bony spicules may damage the median nerve and carpal tunnel syndrome may occur as a late sequela.

367   Fractures of the radial styloid
   A   extend into the wrist joint
   B   typically have an anterior dislocation of the bony fragment
   C   are commonly associated with fractures of the triquetral bone
   D   are commonly associated with fractures of the scaphoid
   E   are commonly associated with dislocation of the wrist joint

368   A transverse fracture of the scaphoid is
   A   the commonest carpal injury
   B   prone to infection
   C   usually seen in young men
   D   prone to avascular necrosis
   E   usually seen on an early scaphoid radiograph

367 A **True**   They require accurate reduction to reduce long term arthritic problems.
     B **False**   Dorsal displacement is usual and large fragments, with the retainable attachment of the brachioradialis muscle, are drawn proximally.
     C **False**   This is usually due to direct trauma and may be associated with other carpal injuries.
     D **False**   This is the commonest carpal injury and must be suspected in any patient with post-traumatic tenderness over the anatomical snuff box even when there are no radiological abnormalities.
     E **False**   Anterior and posterior dislocations of the wrist joint are usually associated with fractures of the corresponding anterior and posterior carpal surfaces of the radius.

368 A **True**   It must be suspected in a young adult with tenderness over the anatomical snuffbox following a fall.
     B **False**   It is rarely compound so infection is not a problem.
     C **True**   This injury is sustained by falling on the outstretched hand. In older patients this same injury produces a Colles' fracture.
     D **True**   Prolonged immobilisation minimises the risk of avascular necrosis and non-union. For this reason plasters are worn until radiological healing is present.
     E **False**   Fractures of the scaphoid are often not seen on the earliest radiographs and the diagnosis must be made clincally (a painful wrist with tenderness in the anatomical snuff box). Reduction is best achieved with the wrist flexed. Repeat radiographs taken 2 weeks after the injury may then demonstrate some local reabsorption of bone around the fracture and thus render it more obvious.

369 In pelvic fractures
   A   avulsion injuries are usually treated by early mobilisation
   B   undisplaced lesions of the ischial or pubic rami are usually
       treated by early mobilisation
   C   extraperitoneal urinary extravasation may be due to damage
       either to the membranous urethra or to the base of the
       bladder
   D   extraperitoneal urinary extravasation may be due to damage
       of the base of the bladder
   E   which are unstable, one half of the pelvis is displaced
       proximally by the flank muscles. Reduction may need 40 to
       50 lb (18 to 23 kg) of traction

370 Dislocation of the hip joint
   A   is most common when the hip is in a neutral position
   B   is usually associated with a fracture of the acetabular rim
   C   usually results in the femoral head coming to lie anteriorly
       over the pubis or obturator externus
   D   may be associated with injuries of the sciatic nerve
   E   may fracture the acetabulum

371 Intracapsular fractures of the upper end of the femur are usually
   A   after major trauma in the young
   B   accompanied by shortening of the leg
   C   accompanied by external rotation of the leg
   D   accompanied by adduction of the leg
   E   treated by internal fixation

369 A **True** These injuries affect the anterior superior and inferior iliac spines and are the result of violent muscle contractions. They do not affect the stability of the pelvis and thus do not require prolonged immobilisation.

   B **True** These injuries are usually due to direct trauma. The stability of the pelvis is not markedly affected and weight bearing can be resumed once the initial pain has subsided.

   C **True** Rupture of the puboprostatic ligament may be
   D **True** associated with tearing of the prostate from the membranous urethra. Bony fragments of the fractured pubis may pierce the bladder.

   E **True** In addition, severe pelvic fractures are accompanied by extensive haemorrhage (often concealed), shock and possible bladder and rectal injuries.

370 A **False** The most common dislocation is a posterior one and this is usually the result of force along the line of the femoral shaft when it is flexed at a right angle as in the sitting position. Thus, motorcyclists suffering a sudden decleration frequently sustain posterior dislocations of the hip.

   B **True** The posterior margin of the rim is most commonly affected.

   C **False** This form of dislocation is occasionally seen but in the common posterior dislocation the head lies posterior to the acetabulum.

   D **True** This serious, and sometimes permanent, disability may complicate posterior dislocation of the hip.

   E **True** This is so in central dislocation and may produce soft tissue damage within the pelvis.

371 A **False** These injuries do occur but the fracture is common in the elderly, particularly women, often after minor trauma.

   B **True** This is the result of the longitudinal pull of the hamstring, rectus femoris and iliopsoas muscles.

   C **True** This is due to the action of iliopsoas acting distal to the fracture.

   D **False** Adductor and abductor muscles are both attached to the distal shaft and their actions are thus counterbalanced.

   E **True** This reduces the incidence of avascular necrosis and subsequent non-union. Internal fixation also speeds up mobilisation in these patients who are commonly quite elderly. Very occasionally undisplaced impacted fractures are treated non-surgically.

372 Extracapsular fractures of the upper end of the femur are
   A   usually subtrochanteric in position
   B   usually subject to avascular necrosis of the head of the
       femur
   C   usually accompanied by internal rotation of the leg
   D   usually treated by internal fixation
   E   rarely comminuted

373 In fractures of the mid-shaft of the femur the
   A   proximal fragment is usually flexed
   B   proximal fragment is usually abducted
   C   distal fragment is usually adducted
   D   common femoral vessels are usually damaged
   E   femoral nerve is often damaged

374 In fractures of the patella
   A   comminution is usual when the fracture has been caused by
       indirect violence
   B   a transverse fracture without displacement is usually treated
       by a plaster cylinder with no direct surgical intervention
   C   aspiration of the knee joint should be avoided
   D   a comminuted fracture is best treated by patella excision and
       replacement by a prosthesis
   E   weight bearing should be avoided for the first week

372 A **False** The fracture most commonly lies between the greater and lesser trochanters, i.e. is an intertrochanteric fracture.

 B **False** In this type of fracture healing is usually uneventful. The major part of the blood supply to the head of the femur comes through capsular vessels which are usually undamaged in extracapsular fractures.

 C **False** These fractures show shortening and external rotation as in the intracapsular variety. In addition, adduction of the leg is present as the adductor muscles act on the distal fragment without the opposition of the glutei which remain attached to the proximal fragment.

 D **True** The most commonly used prostheses include a long plate which is screwed onto the upper femoral shaft and a pin which is inserted into the proximal fragment.

 E **False** Comminution and osteoporosis add to the difficulty of precise reduction.

373 A **True** Since the hip flexors are unopposed by the effect of gravity on the distal leg.

 B **True** The attachment of the glutei muscles to the greater trochanter achieves this and the proximal fragment is usually externally rotated.

 C **True** This is due to the unopposed action of the adductor muscles. The hamstrings and quadriceps also produce some shortening of the leg.

 D **False** Extensive bleeding may occur particularly from the profunda vessels but the main artery and vein are not usually directly involved.

 E **False** On rare occasions the sciatic nerve is damaged.

374 A **False** Transverse fractures are more common and usually produced by acute flexion of the knee. Direct injuries to the patella usually produce comminuted fractures.

 B **True** The fragments may be held together by the capsule of the knee joint.

 C **False** There is frequently a large haemarthrosis present which will require aspiration.

 D **False** Excision is only advisable in very severely comminuted fractures and even if this is necessary no prosthesis is required. Tendon suture provides quite good knee flexion.

 E **False** Provided the knee is maintained in extension, weight bearing can be readily undertaken. Active quadriceps exercise may be started on about the tenth day after the injury.

375 In fractures of the middle third of the tibia and fibula
A   delayed union is common
B   indirect violence usually results in a spiral or oblique fracture line
C   shortening and anterior angulation of the tibia are common
D   comminuted fractures are usually treated by early plating of the tibia
E   the tibial nerve is frequently damaged

376 In injuries of the ankle joint
A   eversion injuries are the most commonly encountered
B   inversion injuries are usually accompanied by a tear of the deltoid ligament
C   there is frequently associated posterior tibial nerve damage
D   the posterior tibial artery is frequently damaged
E   the joint is rendered unstable by rupture of the inferior tibiofibular ligament

375 A **True**   These fractures are frequently compound. There is a relatively poor blood supply to the bones in this region, and interposition of muscle and superadded infection are frequent complications. Therefore the incidence of delayed union is high.

  B **True**   Particularly if a twisting force is imparted to the foot.

  C **True**   The anterior surface of the tibia is unsupported by muscles and no splinting effect occurs.

  D **False** These fractures are usually due to direct injury and are compound. Internal fixation is therefore best avoided.

  E **False** However, neurovascular damage must be looked for in every patient.

376 A **False** The ankle is more unstable in the inverted position.

  B **False** This injury affects the lateral not the medial ligament of the joint.

  C **False** Nerve and vascular complications are exceedingly

  D **False** rare.

  E **True**   This injury requires external or internal fixation for 6 weeks prior to any weight bearing.

18 Orthopaedic surgery

377 In rheumatoid arthritis the

   A principal lesion is an area of fibrinoid necrosis surrounded by fibroblasts

   B synovial membrane characteristically undergoes marked hypertrophy

   C fibrosis in the joint capsule and ligaments produces the main deforming forces in the early stages of the disease

   D permanent deformity in the late stage of the disease is usually due to bone ankylosis

   E radiological signs occur at a late stage in the disease

378 Rheumatoid arthritis

   A is characteristically symmetrical in its involvement of the more proximal joints

   B has an equivalent disease in childhood which is also associated with pericarditis

   C carries a worse prognosis if serological tests (such as the Rose Waaler and Latex tests) are positive

   D is characterised by the pes anserinus deformity

   E is characterised by increased activity within an inflamed joint

379 In rheumatoid arthritis

   A females are affected seven times more commonly than males

   B the onset of the disease is usually in the fourth decade

   C the disease is rapidly progressive in 25 per cent of patients

   D approximately 50 per cent of patients have a remission in the first year

   E the symptoms are least apparent in the morning

377 A **True** These are the characteristic changes of the rheumatoid nodule.

B **True** This feature accounts for the joint swelling and the inflammatory mass which extends over the articular surface (known as the pannus).

C **False** The early deformity is due to the laxity of the diseased capsule and ligaments together with associated muscle spasm.

D **False** Although bone ankylosis does occur it is rare. These permanent deformities are usually due to periarticular fibrosis.

E **False** These are early features. Soft tissue expansion and adjacent osteoporotic changes are characteristic.

378 A **True** The disease starts distally and gradually extends to more proximal joints.

B **True** Still's disease – the childhood equivalent – is also characterised by skin rashes, lymphadenopathy and splenomegaly. The illness usually produces more systemic effects and is more rapid in onset than the adult form.

C **True** These tests are positive in approximately 25 per cent of cases.

D **False** This term has no connection with rheumatoid arthritis (it in fact describes the division of the facial nerve). The proximal interphalangeal joints frequently show, however, a swan neck deformity produced by hyperextension of these joints.

E **False** Complement activity is reduced, supporting the concept of an underlying immune mechanism in the disease.

379 A **False** The increased incidence is approximately 3:1.

B **False** The disease commonly starts in young adults with a peak incidence in the fifth decade.

C **False** Approximately 10 per cent fall into this category.

D **True** But if this does not happen within 3 years it is unlikely to occur.

E **False** Morning stiffness is characteristic and may involve non-inflamed joints as well as those clinically involved in the disease process.

380   Rheumatoid arthritis often has an associated
   A   sacroileitis
   B   photosensitivity
   C   anicteric hepatitis
   D   conjunctivitis
   E   Heberden's nodes

381   Acute osteomyelitis in childhood
   A   is usually the result of compound bony injuries
   B   is characterised by a constant bone pain
   C   characteristically produces necrosis of the periosteum
        overlying the infected bone
   D   is not usually demonstrable radiologically for the first 2
        weeks of the disease
   E   may be demonstrated by scintigraphy within 2 to 3 days of
        onset

382   In tuberculosis of the bone
   A   the local reaction is characterised by extensive new bone
        formation
   B   the metaphysis of a long bone is the commonest site of
        involvement
   C   the infection is usually secondary to a primary focus
        elsewhere in the body
   D   extension of the bone abscess into a joint is common
   E   the presentation is typically severe pain over the end of a
        long bone

380 A **False** This is characteristic of ankylosing spondylitis, about a third of which develop peripheral arthritis.

   B **False** This is a feature of systemic lupus erythematosus. This may present with joint abnormalities but bony erosion is unusual.

   C **False** The jaundice of viral hepatitis may be preceded by peripheral arthralgia and myalgia.

   D **False** Conjunctivitis and urethritis are features of Reiter's syndrome, polyarthritis is also a prominent feature.

   E **False** These are features of osteoarthritis.

---

381 A **False** It is usually haematogenous in origin, arising from foci such as boils, infected tonsils or urinary tract infections. Exogenous infections are more common in the adult form of the disease.

   B **True** A constant pain of increasing severity is present from the earliest stages of the infection.

   C **False** Bone necrosis frequently follows acute osteomyelitis. The dead bone is known as a sequestrum. The overlying periosteum usually survives and forms new subperiosteal bone known as the involucrum which thus often surrounds a subperiosteal abscess.

   D **True** Radiological evidence of bone infection may not be evident until the first subperiosteal new bone appears in 14 to 21 days. Antibiotic treatment must be instituted on clinical grounds as soon as the diagnosis is made.

   E **True** But a negative scan must never delay treatment based on a clinical diagnosis.

---

382 A **False** In bone tuberculosis, osteoporosis and bone lysis is usually present. There is much less tendency to new bone formation than in pyogenic bone infection.

   B **False** The infection nearly always starts in the epiphysis.

   C **True** It is a blood-borne metastatic infection which spreads from primary foci in the lungs, bowel or lymph nodes.

   D **True** This is a consequence of the location of the infection and often results in joint destruction and extension of the abscess into the surrounding soft tissues.

   E **False** The abscesses show few of the classical signs of inflammation and may grow to a large size before presentation.

383 In osteoarthritis of the hip joint
 A the articular cartilage undergoes initial hypertrophy and then becomes hardened and eburnated
 B the joint capsule becomes stretched and lax
 C the leg is usually adducted and externally rotated when the patient lies supine
 D a femoral osteotomy usually helps halt the progress of the disease process
 E associated changes in the ankle joint are rare

384 Osteoarthritis
 A is the commonest arthropathy
 B is characterised by marginal osteophyte formation
 C commonly presents with back pain
 D symptoms are least apparent in the morning
 E commonly produces swelling of the distal interphalangeal joints

385 In Paget's disease of the bone
 A the serum alkaline phosphatase is considerably raised
 B spiral fractures of the femur are common
 C deafness is a characteristic of the later stages of the disease
 D the fibula is typically affected
 E osteogenic sarcoma develops twice as commonly as in unaffected people

383 A **False** The articular cartilage thins and becomes rough; the underlying bone then becomes dense and smooth (eburnated) and cysts usually develop in the perichondral bone.

B **False** The capsule becomes thick and fibrosed. At the extremes of movement some tearing may occur and this gives rise to further fibrosis.

C **True** Some degree of fixed flexion deformity is also commonly present.

D **True** In some cases the joint changes are partly reversed. The operation should be performed before the head of the femur has collapsed. Improvement is unlikely if this has already occurred.

E **True** The shoulder, elbow and wrist joints are also rarely affected.

384 A **True** Some radiological changes present in the majority of people over the age of 55 years and over 30 per cent have some symptoms.

B **True** The increased body loading following cartilage destruction produces remodelling and new bone formation.

C **False** Although spinal changes are common, pain is usually in the weight bearing hip and knee joints.

D **True** Morning joint stiffness is characteristic of rheumatoid arthritis.

E **True** These are present in more than 50 per cent of patients.

385 A **True**

B **False** Though pathological fractures of the femur do occur in this condition, they are usually of the transverse variety and are typically in the subtrochanteric region of the femur.

C **True** The bony thickening and deformity commonly involves the skull and may thus interfere with the transmission of sound vibrations.

D **False** The spine, femur and tibia are the commonest sites of involvement.

E **False** There is a greatly increased rate of osteogenic sarcoma formation in these patients. It is more than 30 times that of the normal population and the tumour appears to be a particularly malignant variety.

386   Dyschondroplasia is characterised by
   A   a large skull with a short base and a snub nose
   B   short stubby fingers (the trident hand)
   C   being inherited as a Mendelian dominant
   D   multiple enchondromata of the fingers and toes
   E   congenital dislocation of the hip

387   Diaphysial aclasis is characterised by
   A   a defect in cartilagenous ossification
   B   multiple fractures and subsequent deformity
   C   blue sclera
   D   being familial in origin
   E   an increased incidence of sarcomatous bone disease

388   Dupuytren's contracture of the palm
   A   is transmitted as a Mendelian dominant
   B   is predominantly seen in men
   C   has an association with glomerulonephritis
   D   which is long-standing, is often associated with secondary
       fibrosis of the interphalangeal joints
   E   extends proximally along the lateral aspect of the hand

386 A **False** These are all features of achondroplasia – typified by
      B **False** the short-limbed circus dwarf. There is frequently a
                   lordosis present.

      C **False**
      D **True**   The disease is also known as multiple
                   enchondromatosis or Ollier's disease. It is due to the
                   failure of ossification of areas of cartilage in the
                   epiphyses.
      E **False** Congenital hip dysplasia is not a feature of the
                   disease.

387 A **True**   The condition is also known as multiple exostosis.
                   Large bony outgrowths appear at the ends of long
                   bones arising from the epiphyseal plate.
      B **False** These features are typical of osteogenesis imperfecta
      C **False** which often presents with frequent fractures
                   following trivial trauma at birth (as a stillbirth) or in
                   later childhood (osteogenesis imperfecta tarda).
      D **True**   It is an autosomal dominant, and commoner in
                   males.
      E **True**   Although sarcomatous changes are rare, the large
                   number of exostoses increase the risk.

388 A **False** There is, however, an inherited predisposition to this
                   disease.
      B **True**   The frequency is 10:1.
      C **False** It is associated with liver disease and chronic
                   alcoholism.
      D **True**   This may necessitate amputation of the digit.
      E **False** The ring and little finger are most frequently
                   involved.

389 In a case of congenital dislocation of the hip
A   the defect cannot be detected until the third week of life
B   there is a defect of the posterior rim of the acetabulum
C   on bilateral hip abduction with the knees flexed there is often limited abduction on the diseased side
D   reduction is sometimes hindered by a tight gluteus minimus muscle
E   splinting of the limbs following reduction should be maintained until the femoral epiphysis returns to its normal density on radiographic examination

390 Slipped femoral epiphyses
A   occur between the ages of 5 and 10 years
B   typically are seen in overweight children
C   are bilateral in 20 per cent of patients
D   are displaced downwards and posteriorly in relation to the neck of the femur
E   are usually associated with dislocation of the femoral head

391 Perthes' disease of the hip
A   is a degenerative disease of the elderly
B   often presents with a fixed flexion deformity of the hip
C   is accompanied by increased joint mobility
D   may, in most cases, be treated non-surgically
E   has a better prognosis when diagnosed in a younger patient

389 A **False** The signs are usually present at birth but checks should be repeated throughout the neonatal visits.

B **False** The acetabular defect is superior, although the dislocation is always posterior. The consistency of this defect is one of the factors supporting the genetic theory of origin (20 per cent familial). Other theories are abnormal intrauterine positioning and capsular laxity due to maternal hormones

C **True** This is the basis of Ortolani's test – the hip often clicking (or jerking) into position to allow further abduction.

D **False** Characteristic causes limiting a closed reduction are a tight psoas muscle, an hour-glass stricture of the capsule, a thick ligamentum teres and an infolding of the superior labrum glenoidale (known as the limbus).

E **False** Reduction should be maintained until the acetabular roof re-forms, which takes 6 to 9 months in those cases diagnosed early.

390 A **False** The age of peak incidence is 10 to 15 years.

B **True** Boys are affected more commonly than girls.

C **True** Careful follow-up is therefore essential.

D **True** A lateral radiograph of the hip joints is therefore the most informative.

E **False** The head remains within the acetabulum.

391 A **False** This is a disease of young children particularly between the ages of 5 and 10 years. Boys are affected four times more frequently than girls. It is thought to be due to an ischaemic necrosis of the epiphysis of the head of the femur.

B **False** The usual presentation is with pain in the hip and a limp. Radiographs may show fragmentation, flattening and increased density of the femoral head.

C **False** Movements are decreased, especially internal rotation and abduction.

D **True** The deformity of the femoral head and thus the long term sequelae are minimised by non-weight-bearing (often for more than 1 year).

E **True** This is probably due to the smaller epiphysis in the young child which has a better chance of being revascularised.

392   Injury to the medial meniscus of the knee joint is
A   often associated with a tear of the quadriceps femoris
B   less common than that of the lateral meniscus
C   often present in cases of locking of the knee
D   characterised by a positive draw sign
E   commonly associated with local tenderness

393   Hallux valgus is commonly associated with
A   a raised medial longitudinal arch
B   clawing of toes
C   a perforating ulcer beneath the head of the first metatarsal
D   reduction of vibration sensation over the tip of the great toe
E   a dry vasodilated foot

394   Idiopathic scoliosis
A   is the most common type of scoliosis
B   usually appears between the ages of 10 and 12 years
C   is more common in boys
D   is sometimes familial
E   is usually painless

395   In benign tumours of cartilage
A   chondromata and osteochondromata occur equally in the two sexes
B   malignant changes occur in 10 per cent of cases of multiple osteochondromata
C   chondromata usually occur in the epiphyses of long bones
D   osteochondromata usually occur in the epiphyses of long bones
E   chondromata frequently present with pathological fractures

392   A   **False**   Quadriceps injuries are sometimes produced by
                      minor trauma and this suggests a pre-existing
                      abnormality of the tendon.
      B   **False**   They are the commonest form of internal
                      derangement of the knee.
      C   **True**   This is highly suggestive of a meniscal tear.
      D   **False**   This abnormality is typical of an injury to a cruciate
                      ligament.
      E   **True**   Tenderness is frequently along the medial joint line
                      corresponding to the site of meniscal damage.

393   A   **False**   These are all features of the neuropathic foot, such as
      B   **False**   in the diabetic. The motor neuropathy affects
      C   **False**   predominantly the small muscles of the foot leaving
      D   **False**   the action of the long flexor tendons unopposed. The
      E   **False**   automatic neuropathy produces a vasodilated foot
                      with absence of sweating.

394   A   **True**   The scoliotic deformity produced is severe in this
                      group (the worst being due to the paralytic form).
      B   **True**   There often is marked deterioration over the
                      following years until the completion of vertebral
                      growth.
      C   **False**   There is a predominance of this condition in girls. It
                      has been suggested that the condition is due to
                      subclinical poliomyelitis but as the latter is equally
                      distributed in both sexes this appears unlikely.
      D   **True**   The familial tendency may indicate a genetic
                      aetiology.
      E   **True**   This is one of the reasons for the insidious onset.

395   A   **True**   But the benign chondroblastoma is commoner in
                      males.
      B   **True**   But this is less common in solitary tumours and
                      occurs rarely in chondroblastomata.
      C   **False**   These tumours are usually present in the metaphysis
                      of long bones, particularly in the bones of the hands
                      and feet.
      D   **False**   These tumours are usually seen in the metaphysis of
                      long bones. Chondroblastomata occur primarily in
                      the epiphyses.
      E   **False**   These are rare.

396   Chordomata

  A   of the base of the skull (spheno-occipital) develop in the remnants of Rathke's pouch
  B   of the sacrococcygeal region develop in the remnants of the neural canal
  C   are characterised radiologically by central rarefaction of the bone and cortical thinning and expansion
  D   are commoner in females than in males
  E   usually present soon after puberty

397   An osteoid osteoma

  A   usually presents in the adult
  B   is most frequently seen in the bones of the upper limb
  C   commonly presents with local pain
  D   demonstrates a small circular band of bony sclerosis surrounding a translucent area on radiographs
  E   is a blood-filled cavity lined with a soft membrane

398   The osteoclastoma (giant cell tumour of bone)

  A   characteristically occurs in the shaft of a long bone
  B   usually occurs before fusion of the epiphyseal plate
  C   may be recognised by the subperiosteal new bone which overlies the tumour and is demonstrable radiologically
  D   is very rarely malignant
  E   characteristically presents as a pathological fracture

396 A **False**   These tumours develop from notochordal remnants
    B **False**   and usually occur at the cephalic or caudal extremity
           of the vertebral column.
    C **False**   The characteristic radiological appearances are
           progressive bone destruction and soft tissue
           swelling.
    D **False**   They are twice as common in males.
    E **False**   Presents usually after the age of 30. The symptoms
           are mainly due to neural involvement.

397 A **False**   It most commonly presents during adolescence.
    B **False**   Any bone may be involved but there is a slight
           predilection for the bones of the lower limb.
    C **True**   Particularly so at night. Local tenderness also occurs.
    D **True**   These are the characteristic radiographic
           appearances of osteoid osteoma and they may be
           confused with those of a chronic pyogenic bone
           abscess.
    E **False**   These are the features of an aneurysmal bone cyst.

398 A **False**   It is almost invariably situated at the end of a bone. It
           can occur in any bone but is rare in flat bones.
    B **False**   The commonest age of presentation is in the third
           and fourth decades.
    C **False**   Radiological characteristics do not include
           subperiosteal new bone. There is cortical expansion
           and thinning, together with rarefaction of the
           underlying bone. The cortex may be totally destroyed
           in the later stages of the disease.
    D **False**   Local recurrence is present in almost half the cases
           after attempted surgical removal and malignant
           change is seen in about 15 per cent. Treatment
           should be by wide excision.
    E **False**   Although these can occur, especially in large
           tumours, they are usually treated before this time.

399   Osteogenic sarcomata
  A   are most frequent in the 10 to 25 year age group
  B   are frequently sited around the knee
  C   readily metastasise via the bloodstream
  D   are frequently surrounded by non-malignant new bone
      formation
  E   when treated by radical surgery have a 50 per cent 5-year
      survival rate

400   The Ewing's sarcoma of bone
  A   is classically a disease of middle age and late years
  B   can be effectively treated by radiotherapy
  C   frequently results in a pathological fracture
  D   usually occurs in the diaphyses of the long bones
  E   does not metastasise

399 A **True**   The majority occur in this age group, exceptions
being those occurring in late life in patients with
Paget's disease of the bone.
B **True**   In the distal femur or proximal tibia. Other common
sites are the proximal humerus and femur, and the
pelvis.
C **True**   Pulmonary metastases are particularly common.
Lymph node metastases are very uncommon.
D **True**   The periosteum overlying an osteogenic sarcoma is
raised by the tumour. This produces the
characteristic radiological appearances of the
overlying periosteum having underneath it a
triangular area of new bone formation (Codman's
triangle). The tumour itself comprises radiating
spicules of new bone formation ('sunray') and
variable degrees of lysis and sclerosis.
E **False**   Radical surgery is usually combined with
preoperative radiotherapy. Not more than 5 to 10 per
cent of patients survive 5 years. Recently there have
been encouraging reports of improved survival
figures after the use of multiple chemotherapy.

400 A **False**   The usual presentation is in infancy and up to the age
of 25 years. It is more frequent in males.
B **False**   Survival varies from a few months to a few years.
Whilst radiotherapy provides some symptomatic
relief, neither this nor surgery is usually curative. The
tumour is often multicentric in origin and adjuvant
chemotherapy has been added to the treatment
protocol with some encouraging improvement in the
results.
C **False**   The most frequent radiographic appearance is of
overlapping layers of new subperiosteal bone
formation, the so called 'onion peel' effect. This new
bone has normal strength; thus pathological
fractures are very uncommon.
D **True**   It is extremely uncommon for any other portion of
the bone to be affected.
E **False**   Although pulmonary metastases do not occur as
frequently as in osteogenic sarcoma, widespread
metastases are common in the terminal stages.

401 Fibrosarcomata of the bone
   A   are the most malignant of bone tumours
   B   most commonly occur in the bones of the tarsus
   C   demonstrate bone destruction with no new bone formation
        on radiograph
   D   usually present with pulmonary metastases
   E   are commonest in the third and fourth decades

402 Chondrosarcomata
   A   which develop in the metaphysis are usually less well
        differentiated than those occurring around the epiphysis
   B   quite commonly invade the neighbouring blood vessels
   C   commonly metastasise to lymph nodes
   D   characteristically present as a pathological fracture
   E   are the commonest malignant tumour of bone

401 A **False** They are slower growing than osteogenic sarcomata and a 5-year survival rate of approximately 25 per cent is frequently reported. Treatment is by radical amputation.

    B **False** The sites of predilection are similar to those of the osteogenic sarcoma, i.e. in the ends of long bones, particularly the femur, tibia and humerus.

    C **True** The absence of radiating bone spiculation distinguishes it from osteogenic sarcoma.

    D **False** The most usual presentation is of a local, painful, progressive swelling around the knee, elbow or shoulder joint and sometimes a pathological fracture.

    E **True** They occur at any age. Tumours associated with Paget's disease present later in life.

---

402 A **True** Metaphyseal tumours often develop from osteochondromata whereas the peripheral tumours are formed of more mature cartilage. These tumours are slightly commoner in males and occur between the ages of 30 to 60 years.

    B **True** Extension into the blood vessels is quite frequent.

    C **False** Metastases are usually seen late in the disease and are blood borne, commonly producing peripheral lung deposits. Lymph node metastases are rare.

    D **False** The commonest presentation is of a painful bony swelling. Tenderness is present, particularly when haemorrhage and extraosseous extension has occurred.

    E **False** Osteogenic sarcomata are commonest and are about twice as common as chondrosarcomata.

19 Neurosurgery

403 Intracranial aneurysms
- **A** are the cause of the vast majority of cases of spontaneous subarachnoid haemorrhage
- **B** usually occur in the third and fourth decade
- **C** are multiple in 20 per cent of cases
- **D** frequently rebleed after an initial haemorrhage
- **E** which have ruptured require surgical treatment which involves clipping of the appropriate middle cerebral artery

404 In head injuries the causes of a rising intracranial pressure include
- **A** intracerebral haemorrhage
- **B** cerebral oedema
- **C** rhinorrhoea
- **D** meningitis
- **E** artificial ventilation

403 A **False** Intracranial aneurysms are the cause of over 50 per cent of spontaneous subarachnoid haemorrhage but the remainder are due to arteriovenous malformations, blood dyscrasias, anticoagulant therapy and hypertension, together with a large group of unknown aetiology.

   B **True** They rarely occur before the age of 20 years and, although slightly commoner in young males, are, overall, commoner in females.

   C **True** These occur at arterial bifurcations around the circle of Willis.

   D **True** This carries with it a higher morbidity and mortality than the first bleed.

   E **False** Surgical treatment where indicated is directed at (i) excluding the aneurysms by clipping it at its neck, (ii) reinforcing its walls with fascia or synthetic material, or (iii) promoting thrombosis by injecting into it or by reducing its blood flow, e.g. by a carotid ligation. Clipping of the middle cerebral artery will usually produce serious neurological complications.

404 A **True** This is one of the three common types of post-traumatic intracranial haemorrhage.

   B **True** This may develop within a few hours and contribute to the mortality of severe cases. It is normally treated by diuretic therapy, fluid restriction and steroids.

   C **False** This and otorrhoea usually subside within a few days. If they persist, craniotomy and some form of surgical repair of the dura is undertaken.

   D **True** This may follow closed as well as open cerebral injuries but it is more common in the latter. Prophylactic antibacterial therapy is indicated in open injuries.

   E **False** Hyperventilation may reduce intracranial pressure due to hypocapnia.

405   In head injuries the signs of an expanding intracranial lesion include
A   a falling level of consciousness
B   a rising pulse rate
C   a falling blood pressure
D   small pupils
E   tachypnoea

406   Following head injuries surgical intervention is usually required for
A   linear skull fractures
B   cerebral oedema
C   depressed skull fractures
D   extradural haemorrhage
E   a decreasing level of consciousness

405 A **True** This is the most important of signs. Ensure that reproducible factors (such as whether or not the patient knows his name, age and address and the manner in which he obeys simple commands) are fully recorded at frequent intervals.

B **False** The reverse is the case, the pulse rate falls and the
C **False** blood pressure rises. These vital signs must be observed at least every 15 minutes until normal stable values are maintained.

D **False** These may be present in the initial stage due to stimulation of the oculomotor nerve but progressive increase in pressure shifts the brain and puts pressure on the oculomotor nerves resulting in pupillary dilatation (small pupils are seen with pontine injuries and these carry a very bad prognosis).

E **False** The respiratory rate falls and may become Cheyne–Stokes in nature.

---

406 A **False** Linear skull fractures demand careful observation of the patient's vital signs in order to detect such complications as haemorrhage or infection. In the absence of these signs they do not require surgery.

B **False** There is no satisfactory surgical cure for post-traumatic cerebral oedema.

C **True** Surgery is required in all but minor depressions over non-vital areas

D **True** This is usually due to damage of the middle meningeal vessels often in association with linear fractures of the temporal bone. Typically the patient loses consciousness at the time of the accident due to concussion. Consciousness then returns (the so-called lucid interval) until increasing intracranial pressure results in a falling of the level of consciousness. Emergency surgery is indicated to evacuate the clot and control the haemorrhage.

E **False** Surgery is undertaken for specific indications and these are greatly facilitated by CT scanning.

407 Head injuries may be complicated by
  A hydrocephalus
  B haematuria
  C epilepsy
  D diabetes insipidus
  E diabetes mellitus

408 Chronic subdural haematomata
  A are common in children
  B have a characteristic angiographic appearance
  C should be treated surgically
  D have a better postoperative prognosis than acute subdural haematomata
  E may present as dementia

409 The characteristic signs of chronically raised intracranial pressure include
  A a bitemporal hemianopia
  B papilloedema
  C epilepsy
  D bradycardia
  E gastrointestinal haemorrhage

407 A **True**   The advent of the CT scanning has revealed that post-traumatic hydrocephalus frequently follows severe head injury. It is due to obstruction of the aqueduct of blood and may require ventricular drainage or an indwelling shunt.

    B **False**   There is no association.

    C **True**   The risks are highest in those who have had a post-traumatic amnesia for more than 24 hours, dural penetration, a missile injury or early epilepsy.

    D **True**   It is fortunately rare but follows pituitary necrosis secondary to trauma or hypoxia.

    E **False**   This is not associated.

408 A **False**   They occur characteristically in the aged and often follow minor injuries. They are rarely associated with skull fractures.

    B **True**   The cortical vessels are displaced from the vault and there is a shift in the midline structures away from the side of the lesion. CT scanning is the primary investigation.

    C **True**   Acute subdural haemorrhage follows severe trauma
    D **True**   and is often bilateral. It is associated with more severe underlying permanent damage to the brain, and has a worse prognosis than the chronic subdural haematoma. The latter should be treated surgically since it is generally associated with very minor underlying cerebral injury and the results are good.

    E **True**   But the diagnosis can be easily missed.

409 A **False**   This characteristically follows pressure on the optic decussation from a pituitary tumour or a suprasellar meningioma.

    B **True**   Papilloedema accompanies a raised intracranial pressure and is not, in its early phase, accompanied by visual symptoms.

    C **True**   This may be grand mal or focal in nature.

    D **True**   This is probably caused by the effect of pressure on the vasomotor centre. Other signs include a falling conscious level and a sixth nerve palsy.

    E **True**   Gastric ulceration may accompany raised intracranial pressure.

410   Fractures of the maxilla
    A cannot usually be demonstrated radiologically for 48 hours
    B are often accompanied by numbness over the upper lip
    C are often accompanied by diplopia
    D rarely require surgical intervention
    E place the airway at particular risk

411   In fractures of the cervical spine
    A the odontoid process is usually damaged by extension injuries
    B at the base of the odontoid process, the odontoid process is carried forward with the atlas
    C non-union of the odontoid is uncommon
    D involving a spinous process, treatment is usually by internal fixation
    E 'halo' fixation should be avoided in incomplete neurological defects

412   Cervical spondylosis
    A is frequent in the fifth decade
    B may present with long tract motor signs
    C commonly presents with loss of sphincter control
    D typically presents with symmetrical sensory loss
    E can present with syncope

410 A **False**   If suitable views are taken the fracture lines will be seen immediately and there will be opacity of the appropriate maxillary sinus.

   B **True**   The infraorbital nerve is usually damaged as the fracture line typically passes through the infraorbital canal.

   C **True**   The fracture may involve the bony attachments of the suspensory ligament of the eye.

   D **False**   Some form of fixation is usually necessary to avoid persistent diplopia, limitation of jaw movement and cosmetic deformity.

   E **True**   In bilateral fractures the maxilla may be displaced posteriorly. Injury must be carefully looked for since it may be masked by extensive oedema.

411 A **False**   The commonest causes are flexion injuries such as occur in violent deceleration or from a blow to the back of the head.

   B **True**   It is maintained in this position by the transverse ligaments of the atlas.

   C **False**   The initial fracture may be painless and difficult to demonstrate but late films will show an area of sclerosis.

   D **False**   These, like fractures of a transverse process, are usually avulsion injuries and require no specific surgery. Active mobilisation should be encouraged once the initial pain has subsided.

   E **False**   The need for fixation is based on spinal stability rather than neuronal damage.

412 A **False**   It is a degenerative disease increasing with age, about 75 per cent of individuals being affected by the age of 70 years.

   B **True**   The differential diagnosis includes multiple sclerosis and neoplasms of the cervical vertebrae and spinal cord.

   C **False**   This is unusual, but common in neoplastic disease of the spinal cord.

   D **False**   Sensory loss is rare and signs are usually asymmetrical.

   E **True**   Sudden neck extension and rotation can compress the vertebral arteries and alter cerebral blood flow.

413   In a patient with a lumbar disc protrusion
A   loss of the knee jerk is characteristic of a second lumbar nerve root lesion
B   loss of dorsiflexion of the great toes indicates a third lumbar nerve root lesion
C   loss of sensation over the sole indicates a fourth lumbar nerve root lesion
D   loss of the ankle jerk indicates a first sacral nerve root lesion
E   a perianal sensory loss indicates a fourth lumbar nerve root lesion

414   Birth injuries involving the fifth and sixth cervical nerve roots of the brachial plexus
A   are known as Klumpke's palsy
B   are rarely followed by full recovery
C   are characterised by the arm being held in the pronated and internally rotated position
D   produce paralysis of the triceps muscle
E   show weakness and wasting of the small muscles of the hand

415   Following a peripheral nerve injury
A   loss of axon continuity is described as neuropraxia
B   the proximal axon undergoes Wallerian degeneration
C   due to gunshot wounds primary nerve repair is desirable
D   delayed suture is best performed 1 week after the injury
E   delayed suture is best performed 3 months after the injury

413 A **False** The knee jerk is mediated via the third and fourth lumbar nerve roots.
     B **False** This useful physical sign indicates a lesion of the fifth lumbar nerve root.
     C **False** The sole is supplied via the first sacral nerve root.
     D **True**
     E **False** The sphincter is supplied by the third sacral nerve root.

414 A **False** This injury is known as Erb's palsy. Klumpke's palsy is a lesion involving the eighth cervical and first thoracic roots of the brachial plexus and is a rare complication of breech delivery.
     B **False** Full recovery is usual in this injury. It is essential to maintain passive movement and to splint the limb to prevent contractions during the recovery phase (recovery is unusual in Klumpke's palsy).
     C **True** The limb is also adducted and splinting should therefore maintain the limb abducted, externally rotated and supinated.
     D **False** This is innervated by the seventh and eighth nerve roots.
     E **False** This is characteristic of first thoracic nerve root injury.

415 A **False** Neuropraxia is temporary impairment of nerve conduction. Loss of axon and nerve continuity are described as axontmesis and neurotmesis respectively.
     B **False** This occurs distal to the injury.
     C **False** Primary nerve repair should only be considered in uncontaminated wounds.
     D **False** The optimal time of nerve repair is 3 to 4 weeks after
     E **False** the injury, providing there is no local infection and the surrounding tissues have healed. The nerve ends can then be mobilised, trimmed of new fibrous tissue and carefully anastomosed.

416   After peripheral nerve section
   A   the axon grows distally at approximately 4 mm/day
   B   the growing end of the nerve can be localised by percussion
   C   primary nerve suture should usually be undertaken
   D   the motor end-plates degenerate after 6 weeks and resuture
         after this period is rarely satisfactory
   E   muscle atrophy is delayed for 6 to 8 weeks

417   In lesions affecting the common peroneal (lateral popliteal) nerve
   A   sensory loss is limited to the dorsal aspect of the first
         interdigital cleft
   B   there is weakness of dorsiflexion of the foot
   C   there is weakness of eversion of the foot
   D   the toes become clawed
   E   there is loss of the ankle jerk

418   Brain abscesses
   A   are usually secondary to sepsis elsewhere in the body
   B   are frequently the consequence of throat infections
   C   are usually multiple
   D   should be treated by antibiotics without surgical drainage
   E   are commonly due to staphyloccocal and streptococcal
         organisms

416 A **False** Although this rate has been described in experimental animals, in the clinical situation recovery rate is not more than 1 to 1.5 mm/day.

    B **True** This is known as Tinnel's sign and refers to the paraesthesia produced over the growing nerve end in response to slight trauma.

    C **False** Except in the rare instances of clean division (e.g. accidental surgical division of the nerve) resuture is best left for about 3 weeks when the damaged area is clearly demarcated and local contamination has subsided.

    D **False** Motor endplate degeneration takes a number of months to occur.

    E **False** Disuse atrophy is of early onset and requires active physiotherapy until re-innervation occurs.

417 A **False** This is the area of sensory loss associated with lesions of the anterior tibial nerve. Involvement of the common peroneal nerve gives rise to sensory loss over the lateral aspect of the leg and the dorsum of the foot.

    B **True** The patient suffers from foot drop and walks with a

    C **True** high stepping gait on the affected side.

    D **False** This is seen in lesions of the tibial (medial popliteal) nerve due to paralysis of the intrinsic muscles of the foot.

    E **False** This is innervated by the tibial nerve.

418 A **True** Infection in the pleural or peritoneal cavity is the usual site of origin in the USA but infection of the paranasal air spaces or chronic suppurative otitis media are common causes in the UK.

    B **False** Since abscesses in the frontal or parietal lobes account for more than 50 per cent of brain abscesses.

    C **False** Multiple abscesses are rare and occur usually in immune suppressed patients.

    D **False** Surgical drainage with appropriate antibiotic therapy is almost always required. It should be monitored by frequent CT scans. In the few cases when diagnosis occurs at the stage of cerebritis with no pus, success has followed monitoring with CT scans and antibiotic treatment.

    E **True** Anaerobic organisms account for approximately 50 per cent of cases, multiple organisms for 5 per cent and no organisms are found in 20 per cent of cases.

419 Brain tumours

    A in the adult are most commonly glioblastomata multiforme

    B in children are most commonly medulloblastomata

    C of childhood are most commonly found in the posterior cranial fossa

    D which arise extracerebrally are most commonly acoustic neuromata

    E are metastases in approximately 20 per cent of cases

420 Meningiomas

    A are common in females

    B are frequently seen in children

    C frequently occur along the sphenoid ridge

    D derive their blood supply mostly through the internal carotid artery

    E typically reach their maximum size within 9 months of onset

419 A **True**   These are highly malignant, showing rapid growth
          and marked invasiveness.
     B **True**   These are by far the most common and, together
     C **True**   with other posterior fossa tumours such as the
          cerebellar astrocystoma, make up the vast majority
          of childhood intracranial tumours.
     D **False** Meningiomas are the commonest extracerebral
          tumour followed by acoustic neuromas and pituitary
          tumours.
     E **False** This incidence is approximately 50 per cent.

420 A **True**   As are intracranial neuromata, whereas most glial
          tumours are commoner in males.
     B **False** Childhood meningiomas make up only a few per cent
          of cases.
     C **True**   Parasagittal meningiomas are also common.
     D **False** The external carotid artery is the source.
     E **False** They are slow growing and may take a number of
          years to present.

20 Self-assessment examination

1 **The problems of a diabetic foot are mediated by**
   A   large vessel arterial disease
   B   neuropathy
   C   altered inflammatory response
   D   postphlebitic syndrome
   E   ketoacidosis

2 **Acute lower limb ischaemia is accompanied by**
   A   motor paralysis
   B   sparing of foot pulses
   C   hyperaesthesia
   D   sweating of the foot
   E   autonomic neuropathy

3 **Raynaud's syndrome may be associated with**
   A   ingestion of ergot-containing drugs
   B   polyarteritis nodosa
   C   cervical ribs
   D   malignant disease
   E   acute infections

4 **In intracapsular fractures of the head of the femur**
   A   there is usually leg lengthening
   B   the leg is usually externally rotated
   C   the leg is usually adducted
   D   the treatment is usually by internal fixation
   E   the head is subject to avascular necrosis

5 **Injuries of the ankle are commonly**
   A   associated with tibial nerve injury
   B   associated with posterior tibial artery injury
   C   inversion injuries
   D   accompanied by fractures of the talus
   E   treated by internal fixation

6 **In rheumatoid arthritis**
  A there is usually symmetrical involvement of the proximal joints
  B the bony surfaces become ebernated
  C ligamentous laxity occurs at an early phase
  D bony ankylosis is a common end point
  E there is marked synovial hypertrophy

7 **An acute increase of intracranial pressure is accompanied by**
  A a raised blood pressure
  B hypothermia
  C tachycardia
  D erosion of the dorsum sellae
  E papilloedema

8 **A chronic rise in intracranial pressure is accompanied by**
  A papilloedema
  B epilepsy
  C homonymous hemianopia
  D tachycardia
  E hypothermia

9 **In lesions of the lateral popliteal nerve**
  A the toes become clawed
  B there is weakness of inversion of the foot
  C there is sensory loss over the dorsum of the foot
  D the ankle jerk is lost
  E there is weakness of dorsiflexion of the foot

10 **Incisional hernias**
  A are usually para-umbilical in position
  B usually occur in males
  C are usually covered by two muscle layers
  D rarely strangulate
  E are usually related to anaemia

11 **Urinary tract injuries**
  A are usually accompanied by haematuria
  B involving the kidney require urgent surgery
  C involving the bladder are usually intraperitoneal
  D involving the urethra are commonly due to road traffic accidents
  E often present with renal failure

12 The spleen
A   is the commonest abdominal organ to be injured
B   is subject to delayed rupture following blunt trauma
C   can usually be preserved after blunt injury
D   which is injured produces buttock pain
E   is protected from injury by its posterior position

13 Malignant melanoma
A   is rare in black races
B   usually presents between the ages of 20 to 30 years
C   frequently arises in junctional naevi
D   has the best prognosis when occurring in the lower limb
E   should be suspected when bleeding occurs in any pigmented lesion

14 Squamous carcinoma of the skin
A   is common in black races
B   rarely metastasises via the bloodstream
C   is usually best managed by surgical excision
D   commonly arises in a pre-existing papilloma
E   is most common in early adult life

15 Fibroadenomas of the breast
A   are rare in teenagers
B   are usually well circumscribed lumps
C   usually present as a painful lump
D   resolve spontaneously
E   can be diagnosed on needle aspiration

16 Typical radiological features of hyperparathyroidism include
A   nephrocalcinosis
B   bone cysts
C   increased subperiosteal bone density
D   gallstones
E   rib fractures

17 Phaeochromocytomas
A   arise from splenic mesoderm
B   are often multiple
C   present with bradycardia
D   present with abdominal striae
E   are subject to fulminating septicaemia

18 Typical features of Cushing's syndrome include
A   bradycardia
B   hypokalaemia
C   hypertension
D   diabetes insipidus
E   polycythaemia

19 Gastric cancer is commonly

A found in pre-existing polyps
B in the fundal region
C an adenocarcinoma
D an ulcerating lesion
E preceded by pancreatitis

20 Duodenal ulcers are

A frequently sited in the second part of the duodenum
B typically associated with pancreatitis
C typically associated with gallstones
D equally distributed between the sexes
E characterised by postprandial pain

21 Crohn's disease

A is associated with finger clubbing
B has an equal sex incidence
C is associated with arthralgia
D is limited to the mucosa
E commonly presents with colicky abdominal pain

22 Colonic polyps

A become malignant in 50 per cent of cases
B may be inherited as a Mendelian recessive
C are usually villous adenomas
D commonly present with intussusception
E commonly present with intestinal obstruction

23 Cancers of the right colon

A have an 80 per cent 5-year mortality
B usually present with intestinal obstruction
C often present with an abdominal mass
D may present with anaemia
E are subject to anastomotic recurrence

24 Fresh rectal bleeding is typical of

A rectal cancer
B anal fissure
C sigmoid volvulus
D anticoagulant overdose
E anal fistula

25 Primary liver cancer

A often presents with ascites
B is commoner in patients with cirrhosis
C produces a raised serum alphafetoprotein
D may be related to the female contraceptive pill
E is commoner in Polish immigrants

26 Acute cholecystitis

A   is generally an indication for urgent cholecystectomy
B   usually presents as biliary colic
C   is usually associated with a mild pancreatitis
D   rarely occurs in the absence of gallstones
E   is characterised by a pyrexia in the early hours of the disease

27 Gallstones

A   in the Western world are predominantly formed of cholesterol
B   are commoner in males
C   occur in about 15% of adults over the age of 40 years
D   are a supersaturate of bile acids
E   can usually be broken up using transcutaneous lasers

28 Massive blood transfusions may be complicated by

A   hyperkalaemia
B   hypocalcaemia
C   leucopenia
D   hepatic coma
E   hypothermia

29 In major burns

A   fluid replacement is not usually necessary in a burn of less than 25 per cent body surface area
B   the maximum fluid losses are between 12 and 24 hours after the injury
C   fluid requirements are higher for partial than full thickness injuries
D   patients are in a positive nitrogen balance after the first 24 hours post burn
E   the patient has an increased resistance to septicaemia

30 Wound healing is impaired

A   in polycythaemia
B   during steroid therapy
C   by infection
D   during antibiotic therapy
E   in hypoproteinaemia

31 Thromboangitis obliterans

A   involves medium sized arteries of the limb
B   may present with superficial venous thrombosis
C   is almost exclusively a male disease
D   is very rare in non-smokers
E   is a panarteritis

32 The spermatic cord

A is invested by the transverse abdominus muscle
B contains the iliolumbar nerve
C transmits direct inguinal herniae
D contains the testicular artery
E contains the pudendal nerve

33 Seminoma of the testis

A commonly has a positive Aschheim-Zondak pregnancy test
B usually presents as a painless testicular lump
C commonly metastasises to the pre-aortic nodes
D is very sensitive to radiotherapy
E rarely metastasises via the bloodstream

34 In Paget's disease of the bone there is

A a substantial rise in serum acid phosphatase
B fibrosis of joint capsules
C increased skull density
D a predisposition to femoral fractures
E an increased risk of osteogenic sarcoma formation

35 In cases of congenital dislocation of the hip there is

A a superior defect in the acetabulum
B limited abduction
C an abnormal femoral epiphysis
D a predisposition to an hour-glass capsular deformity
E an attenuated ligamentum teres

36 Perthes' disease of the hip

A is commonest between the ages of 5 and 10 years
B usually presents with a fixed flexion deformity
C is characterised by necrosis of the epiphysis
D is usually managed surgically
E is bilateral in 30 per cent of cases

37 In Erb's palsy there is

A rarely complete recovery
B wasting of the small muscles of the hand
C weakness of elbow flexion
D weakness of elbow extension
E sensory loss along the medial border of the forearm

38 Following peripheral nerve injuries the

A axon grows distally at approximately 1 mm per day
B motor end-plate degenerates within 4 weeks
C optimal time for delayed suture is 3 to 4 weeks
D proximal axon degenerates
E growing end of the nerve can be localised by percussion

39 Characteristic signs of crush injuries to the chest include

A pulsus paradoxus
B facial pallor
C subconjunctival haemorrhage
D cardiac arrhythmias
E abdominal distension

40 Faeculent vomiting is characteristic of

A an upper gastrointestinal bleed
B gastrocolic fistulae
C large bowel obstruction
D chronic appendicitis
E gastroduodenal perforation

41 A perforated duodenal ulcer is usually

A in males
B in the second part of the duodenum
C insidious in onset
D accompanied by board-like abdominal rigidity
E preceded by exacerbation of ulcer symptoms

42 Acute appendicitis

A is commoner in females
B presents with pain around the umbilicus
C is commonest under the age of 15 years
D is usually accompanied by microscopic haematuria
E is commonly associated with a mild pyrexia

43 Paget's disease of the breast

A usually presents with bilateral eczema
B is associated with an underlying neoplasm in approximately 80 per cent of patients
C is an indication of metastatic breast disease
D has characteristic clear, vacuolated cells
E is an intraduct malignancy

44 Breast cancer

A is the second commonest female neoplasm in the United Kingdom
B often presents with a clear nipple discharge.
C is reduced after premenopausal oophorectomy
D can be diagnosed clinically in approximately 90 per cent of cases
E is bilateral in 20 per cent of cases

45 Skin changes indicating inoperable breast cancer include
- A tethering
- B ulceration
- C oedema
- D eczema
- E pigmentation

46 Neuroblastomas
- A often secrete adrenaline precursors
- B rarely metastasise to bone
- C usually arise within the kidney
- D are the commonest solid tumour of infancy
- E usually move freely with respiration

47 Salivary tumours
- A are most commonly sited in the parotid gland
- B commonly produce sialectasis
- C are commonly associated with calculus formation
- D are usually cylindromata
- E typically present with facial pain

48 Cancer of the tongue
- A is typically an adenocarcinoma
- B metastasises early to lymph nodes
- C is commoner in meat eaters
- D is associated with alcoholism
- E has an equal sex distribution

49 Tumours of the small bowel
- A are usually adenocarcinomas
- B are most commonly located in the appendix
- C may present with flushing of the upper parts of the body
- D may be an inherited disorder
- E commonly present with gastrointestinal haemorrhage

50 Chronic radiation bowel injury
- A may present with malabsorption
- B produces extensive mucosal sloughing
- C usually affects the terminal ileum
- D frequently presents with intestinal obstruction
- E produces a progressive vasculitis

51 Meckel's diverticulum
- A is sited at the jejuno-ileal junction
- B may present with gastrointestinal haemorrhage
- C most commonly presents as diverticulitis
- D is devoid of the outer circular layer of muscle wall
- E may communicate with the perineum

52   Haemorrhoids commonly present with
A   pruritus ani
B   fresh rectal bleeding
C   alteration in bowel habit
D   acute anal pain
E   perianal abscess formation

53   An anal fissure commonly presents with
A   pruritus ani
B   perianal pain
C   fresh rectal bleeding
D   alteration in bowel habit
E   perianal abscess formation

54   Rectal prolapse commonly presents
A   in psychiatric institutions
B   post-haemorrhoidectomy
C   with acute anal pain
D   with perianal infection
E   in infants

55   Stones in the common bile duct
A   may produce a prolongation of bleeding time
B   are usually accompanied by progressing jaundice
C   are present in approximately 50 per cent of patients with cholecystitis
D   usually present with a long history of dyspepsia
E   invariably arise in the gallbladder

56   Biliary obstruction
A   frequently produces a biliary fistula
B   may be associated with rigors
C   is commonly due to carcinoma of the common bile duct
D   carries a very high mortality rate
E   is characterised by a rise in serum alkaline phosphatase

57   Hypersplenism typically
A   results in polycythaemia
B   produces thrombocytopenia
C   may accompany portal hypertension
D   produces increased erythropoiesis
E   is improved by splenectomy

58 Tetanus

A may have an incubation period of greater than 20 days
B can be prevented by active immunisation immediately post-injury
C has a better prognosis when the symptoms appear soon after the injury
D is usually produced by *Clostridium perfringens*
E prophylaxis includes antibiotic therapy

59 Small bowel fistulae

A commonly give rise to a metabolic alkalosis
B usually heal spontaneously
C usually have a raised serum bilirubin
D usually produce a rise in serum potassium
E are a common complication following small bowel tumour resection

60 Carcinoma of the bladder

A is usually squamous in origin
B most frequently occurs in the region of the trigone
C is more common in heavy smokers
D usually presents with painful haematuria
E is effectively treated by local surgical resection

61 Benign prostatic enlargement

A is due to enlargement of the periphery of the gland
B usually presents with haematuria
C is effectively managed by hormonal therapy
D typically occurs over the age of 50 years
E is a premalignant condition

62 Carcinoma of the prostate usually

A is an adenocarcinoma
B commences in the middle lobe
C metastasises to the liver
D produces a rise in serum acid phosphatase
E presents early with lower urinary tract symptoms

63 Chondromata are

A commoner in males
B undergo malignant change in 10 per cent of cases
C occur in the epiphysis of long bones
D are common in the hands and feet
E commonly present with local pain

64 Osteoclastomas

A typically occur in flat bones
B are rarely malignant
C are characterised by cortical expansion on a radiograph
D are commonest in the third and fourth decades
E can usually be controlled with chemotherapy

65 Intracranial aneurysms

A account for approximately 50 per cent of cases of spontaneous subarachnoid haemorrhage
B are multiple in 20 per cent of cases
C occur predominantly around the circle of Willis
D frequently re-bleed
E can be effectively managed by induced hypotension

66 A spontaneous pneumothorax

A can be diagnosed by needle aspiration
B can be treated by pleurectomy
C is often treated by lung resection
D is usually associated with tuberosclerosis
E is best diagnosed on a supine chest radiograph

67 Benign tumours of the bronchus

A have a malignant potential
B commonly produce bronchiectasis
C are usually cylindromas
D are closely linked with pipe smoking
E occur predominantly in males

68 Cancer of the bronchus

A has an equal sex incidence
B is usually squamous in origin
C is usually sited in the proximal bronchial tree
D usually presents with a brisk haemoptysis
E may present with the carcinoid syndrome

69 Urgent appendicectomy is indicated for

A a gangrenous appendix
B an adult appendix abscess
C mesenteric adenitis
D Crohn's disease
E acute appendicitis

70 Bad prognostic signs of acute pancreatitis are

A hypocalcaemia
B leucopenia
C the presence of gallstones
D previous attacks
E low back pain

71 **In intestinal obstruction**
   A nasogastric suction should be avoided preoperatively
   B central abdominal distension is characteristic of large bowel involvement
   C there is increased intestinal absorption proximal to the level of obstruction
   D the luminal gas proximal to the obstruction is predominantly carbon dioxide
   E vomiting is an early feature of malignancy

72 **Characteristic features of hyperthyroidism include**
   A lid retraction
   B chemosis
   C visible infrapupillary sclera
   D diarrhoea
   E heat intolerance

73 **In the treatment of hyperthyroidism antithyroid drugs**
   A can usually be withdrawn after 6 months
   B cross the placental barrier
   C are contraindicated in the aged
   D are excreted in breast milk
   E cannot be followed immediately by radioactive iodine

74 **A multinodular goitre**
   A is a premalignant condition
   B may be due to iodine deficiency
   C is associated with regional lymph node enlargement
   D usually indicates reduced secretion of tri-iodothyronine
   E is commonest in males

75 **Oesophageal achalasia**
   A can be diagnosed on mucosal biopsy
   B usually present with dysphagia
   C is linked with a defect of Auerbach's plexus
   D is transmitted as a genetic dominant
   E is associated with peptic ulceration

76 **Peptic oesophagitis is typically associated with**
   A anaemia
   B progressive dysphagia
   C vitamin B_{12} deficiency
   D koilonychia
   E atrophic oral mucosa

77 Para-oesophageal hiatus herniae

A are usually accompanied by oesophagitis
B are frequently associated with gastric ulceration
C rarely occur before middle age
D have a malignant potential
E pass through a defect to the right of the oesophageal opening in the diaphragm

78 Colonic diverticular disease

A is usually asymptomatic
B is commonest in the fourth decade
C may present with severe rectal bleeding
D predominates in the sigmoid colon
E is premalignant

79 Ulcerative colitis is accompanied by

A loss of haustral patterns on barium enema
B pseudopolyposis in the early phase of the disease
C thumb printing of the mucosa on barium enema
D extensive fibrosis of the colonic wall
E ulceration of the ileum

80 Crohn's disease of the rectum is

A frequently associated with anal fissures
B usually accompanied by colonic involvement
C accompanied by extensive submucosal fibrosis
D produces a diffuse granular proctitis
E typified by pseudopolyposis

81 Anal cancer

A is usually of squamous variety
B commonly presents with anal pain
C is associated with haemorrhoids
D spreads to the para-aortic nodes
E can usually be treated by abdominoperineal resection of the rectum

82 Normal bile

A is secreted at the rate of 600 to 800 ml per day
B secretion is reduced after a cholecystectomy
C contains conjugated urobilinogen
D contains no adrenaline
E contains cholecystokinin

83 Bilirubin is
  A conjugated in the liver
  B the breakdown product of haemoglobin
  C partly excreted from the liver as urobilinogen
  D synthesised from cholesterol
  E combined with glucuronic acid in the liver

84 Acute pancreatitis is characterised by a
  A reduction of gut sounds
  B history of gallstones
  C reduction in urinary creatinine
  D raised urinary diastase
  E history of alcoholism

85 The Zollinger-Ellison syndrome is
  A produced by parietal cell neoplasia
  B associated with hyperthyroidism
  C commonly produced by a malignant tumour
  D frequently accompanied by duodenal ulceration
  E characterised by a high serum amylase

86 Cancer of the pancreas
  A commonly occurs in the tail
  B is closely linked with cigarette smoking
  C frequently presents with acute pancreatitis
  D has a raised serum calcium
  E is usually amenable to surgical excision and cure

87 Adenocarcinoma of the kidney typically
  A presents with a pyrexia
  B presents with a leucocytosis
  C spreads along the renal artery
  D metastasises to the liver
  E presents with cannon ball lung metastases

88 Non-union is often seen in fractures of the
  A radiocarpal joint
  B shaft of the fibula
  C talus
  D scaphoid bone
  E condyle of the mandible

89 In fractures of the clavicle
  A the brachial plexus is frequently damaged
  B the injury is usually due to a fall on the outstretched hand
  C the proximal fragment is elevated
  D internal fixation is rarely required
  E the distal fragment is externally rotated

90 In fractures of the surgical neck of the humerus the

   A fragments are usually impacted
   B pectoral nerves are often damaged
   C radial nerve is often damaged
   D distal fragment is usually adducted
   E fracture line is intracapsular

91 In a Colles' fracture the distal radial fragment is

   A usually impacted
   B dorsally angulated
   C ulnar deviated
   D ventrally displaced
   E torn from the intra-articular triangular disc

92 Dislocation of the shoulder joint

   A is commonest in children
   B usually occurs when the arm is in the adducted position
   C commonly displaces the head of the humerus posteriorly
   D frequently damages the median nerve
   E frequently damages the radial nerve

93 Pulmonary embolism

   A is demonstrable at postmortem in 60 per cent of individuals
      over 60 years old
   B is usually of the paradoxical variety
   C can usually be diagnosed on a chest radiograph
   D is commoner in women
   E is particularly common after thyroid surgery

94 An inguinal hernia

   A is usually transilluminable
   B will usually regress spontaneously
   C in a young adult is usually indirect
   D emerges through the superficial inguinal ring
   E emerges lateral to the symphysis pubis

95 Femoral herniae

   A lie adjacent to the femoral nerve
   B emerge medial to the pubic tubercle
   C are lateral to the femoral vein
   D emerge through the saphenous opening
   E pass posterior to the inguinal ligament

96 High intestinal obstruction typically produces

   A metabolic alkalosis
   B hyperkalaemia
   C hypercalcaemia
   D vomiting in the early phase
   E suprapubic pain

97 **Colonic diverticular disease**
   A can usually be diagnosed on sigmoidoscopy
   B often presents with abdominal colic
   C frequently presents with faecal peritonitis
   D is uncommon before the age of 65 years
   E frequently has associated haematuria

98 **The complications of tracheostomy include**
   A laryngeal stenosis
   B aortic arch erosion
   C tracheo-oesophageal fistula
   D erosion of the right brachiocephalic vein
   E tracheal stenosis

99 **Thyroid cancer**
   A rarely presents as a solitary nodule
   B is often accompanied by a bruit
   C is usually of the undifferentiated form
   D usually presents as a hot nodule on an isotope scan
   E occasionally presents with Cushingoid features

100 **Papillary carcinoma of the thyroid**
   A is usually multifocal in origin
   B usually occurs under the age of 25 years
   C can be effectively treated by a thyroid suppressing drug
   D usually spreads via the bloodstream
   E has an equal incidence in both sexes

101 **Typical presenting features of primary hyperparathyroidism include**
   A cardiac arrhythmias
   B muscle weakness
   C diarrhoea
   D weight gain
   E calcinosis cutis

102 **Cancer of the oesophagus**
   A is rarely squamous in origin
   B presents with progressive dysphagia
   C is usually in the middle third
   D is most common in males
   E rarely spreads via the bloodstream

103 **Benign gastric ulcers are more frequent**
   A around 50 years of age
   B in males
   C in the lower social classes
   D than gastric malignancy
   E on the greater than on the lesser curvature of the stomach

104 Gastric cancer is commoner in
A   patients with gastric hyperacidity
B   patients with duodenal ulcers
C   higher social classes
D   females
E   rural areas

105 Ischaemic colitis
A   commonly involves the hepatic flexure
B   may present with late strictures
C   often presents with fresh rectal bleeding
D   is typified by pseudopolyposis
E   produces a diffuse granular proctitis

106 A large bowel volvulus
A   is predominantly encountered in Western Europe
B   usually involves the transverse colon
C   is common in athletes
D   may be reduced non-surgically
E   presents with asymmetrical abdominal distension

107 Hirschsprung's disease
A   usually presents in the young adult
B   is due to submucosal fibrosis
C   may be diagnosed on barium enema
D   can usually be managed conservatively
E   is typified by pseudopolyposis

108 Typical features of chronic liver failure include
A   palmar erythema
B   raised creatinine phosphokinase
C   calcinosis cutis
D   scleroderma
E   raised glutamic pyruvic transaminase

109 Ascites typically accompanies
A   hyperalbuminaemia
B   increased aldosterone secretion
C   raised 5-hydroxyindoleacetic acid levels
D   hypovolaemia
E   hypocalcaemia

110 Bleeding oesophageal varices
A   are due to extra-hepatic causes in the majority of cases
B   can usually be controlled long term with a Sengstaken tube
C   usually present in the third decade
D   are usually accompanied by hypokalaemia
E   should be treated with hypertonic saline infusions

111 The normal adult
- **A** requires 50 mEq/day of potassium
- **B** requires 100 mEq/day of sodium
- **C** has an extracellular pH of 7.1 to 7.3
- **D** requires 70 g/day of protein
- **E** has a plasma volume of 5 litres

112 Postoperative anuria
- **A** is defined as less than 500 ml of urine per day
- **B** requires a fluid intake restriction to 1.5 litres per day
- **C** usually produces a metabolic acidosis
- **D** is usually accompanied by hypokalaemia
- **E** is usually accompanied by hyponatraemia

113 Hypovolaemic shock
- **A** is accompanied by an increase in central venous pressure
- **B** may accompany generalised peritonitis
- **C** is usually accompanied by metabolic alkalosis
- **D** results in an impaired cellular oxygenation
- **E** typically presents with a decreased pulmonary capillary permeability

ANSWERS

1	**A** True	**B** True	**C** True	
	D False	**E** False		
2	**A** True	**B** False	**C** False	
	D False	**E** True		
3	**A** True	**B** True	**C** True	
	D True	**E** False		
4	**A** False	**B** True	**C** False	
	D True	**E** True		
5	**A** False	**B** False	**C** True	
	D False	**E** False		
6	**A** True	**B** False	**C** True	
	D False	**E** True		
7	**A** True	**B** False	**C** False	
	D False	**E** True		
8	**A** True	**B** True	**C** False	
	D False	**E** False		
9	**A** False	**B** False	**C** True	
	D False	**E** True		
10	**A** False	**B** False	**C** False	
	D True	**E** False		
11	**A** True	**B** False	**C** False	
	D True	**E** False		
12	**A** True	**B** True	**C** False	
	C False	**E** False		
13	**A** True	**B** False	**C** True	
	D True	**E** True		
14	**A** False	**B** True	**C** True	
	D False	**E** False		
15	**A** False	**B** True	**C** False	
	D False	**E** True		
16	**A** True	**B** True	**C** False	
	D False	**E** True		
17	**A** False	**B** True	**C** False	
	D False	**E** False		
18	**A** False	**B** False	**C** True	
	D False	**E** True		
19	**A** True	**B** False	**C** True	
	E False	**E** False		
20	**A** False	**B** False	**C** False	
	D False	**E** False		
21	**A** True	**B** True	**C** True	
	D False	**E** True		
22	**A** False	**B** False	**C** False	
	D False	**E** False		
23	**A** False	**B** False	**C** True	
	D True	**E** True		
24	**A** True	**B** True	**C** True	
	D False	**E** False		
25	**A** True	**B** True	**C** True	
	D False	**E** False		
26	**A** False	**B** True	**C** False	
	D True	**E** False		
27	**A** True	**B** False	**C** True	
	D False	**E** False		
28	**A** True	**B** True	**C** False	
	D True	**E** True		
29	**A** False	**B** False	**C** False	
	D False	**E** False		
30	**A** False	**B** True	**C** True	
	D False	**E** True		

| 31 | A True | B True | C True |
| | D True | E False | |

| 32 | A False | B False | C False |
| | D True | E False | |

| 33 | A False | B True | C False |
| | D True | E True | |

| 34 | A False | B False | C True |
| | D True | E True | |

| 35 | A True | B True | C False |
| | D True | E False | |

| 36 | A True | B False | C True |
| | D False | E False | |

| 37 | A False | B False | C True |
| | D False | E False | |

| 38 | A True | B False | C True |
| | D False | E True | |

| 39 | A True | B False | C True |
| | D True | E False | |

| 40 | A False | B False | C False |
| | D False | E False | |

| 41 | A True | B False | C False |
| | D True | E True | |

| 42 | A False | B True | C False |
| | D False | E True | |

| 43 | A False | B False | C False |
| | D True | E True | |

| 44 | A True | B False | C True |
| | D False | E False | |

| 45 | A False | B False | C False |
| | D False | E False | |

| 46 | A True | B False | C False |
| | D True | E False | |

| 47 | A True | B False | C False |
| | D True | E False | |

| 48 | A False | B True | C False |
| | D True | E False | |

| 49 | A False | B True | C True |
| | D True | E False | |

| 50 | A True | B False | C True |
| | D True | E True | |

| 51 | A False | B True | C False |
| | D False | E False | |

| 52 | A True | B True | C False |
| | D False | E False | |

| 53 | A True | B True | C True |
| | D False | E False | |

| 54 | A True | B False | C False |
| | D False | E True | |

| 55 | A True | B False | C False |
| | D True | E False | |

| 56 | A False | B True | C False |
| | D True | E True | |

| 57 | A False | B True | C True |
| | D True | E True | |

| 58 | A True | B False | C False |
| | D False | E True | |

| 59 | A False | B True | C False |
| | D False | E False | |

| 60 | A False | B True | C True |
| | D False | E True | |

| 61 | A False | B False | C False |
| | D True | E False | |

| 62 | A True | B False | C False |
| | D True | E False | |

63	**A** True	**B** False	**C** False
	D True	**E** False	

64	**A** False	**B** False	**C** True
	D True	**E** False	

65	**A** True	**B** True	**C** True
	D True	**E** False	

66	**A** False	**B** True	**C** False
	D False	**E** False	

67	**A** True	**B** True	**C** False
	D False	**E** False	

68	**A** False	**B** True	**C** True
	D False	**E** False	

69	**A** True	**B** False	**C** False
	D False	**E** True	

70	**A** True	**B** False	**C** False
	D False	**E** False	

71	**A** False	**B** False	**C** False
	D False	**E** False	

72	**A** True	**B** True	**C** True
	D True	**E** True	

73	**A** False	**B** True	**C** False
	D True	**E** False	

74	**A** False	**B** True	**C** False
	D False	**E** False	

75	**A** False	**B** True	**C** True
	D False	**E** False	

76	**A** True	**B** False	**C** True
	D False	**E** False	

77	**A** False	**B** True	**C** True
	D False	**E** False	

78	**A** True	**B** False	**C** True
	D True	**E** False	

79	**A** True	**B** False	**C** False
	D False	**E** False	

80	**A** True	**B** True	**C** False
	D True	**E** False	

81	**A** True	**B** True	**C** False
	D False	**E** True	

82	**A** True	**B** False	**C** False
	D False	**E** False	

83	**A** True	**B** True	**C** False
	D False	**E** True	

84	**A** True	**B** True	**C** False
	D True	**E** True	

85	**A** False	**B** False	**C** True
	D True	**E** False	

86	**A** False	**B** False	**C** False
	D False	**E** False	

87	**A** True	**B** False	**C** False
	D False	**E** True	

88	**A** False	**B** False	**C** True
	D True	**E** False	

89	**A** False	**B** True	**C** True
	D True	**E** False	

90	**A** True	**B** False	**C** False
	D False	**E** False	

91	**A** True	**B** True	**C** False
	D False	**E** False	

92	**S** False	**B** False	**C** False
	D False	**E** False	

93	**A** True	**B** False	**C** False
	D False	**E** False	

94	**A** False	**B** False	**C** True
	D True	**E** True	

95	**A** False	**B** False	**C** False
	D True	**E** True	

96	**A** True	**B** False	**C** False
	D True	**E** False	

97	A False	B True	C False
	D False	E False	

98	A False	B False	C False
	D False	E True	

99	A False	B False	C False
	D False	E False	

100	A True	B False	C False
	D False	E False	

101	A False	B True	C False
	D False	E False	

102	A False	B True	C False
	D True	E True	

103	A True	B True	C True
	D True	E False	

104	A False	B False	C False
	D False	E False	

105	A False	B True	C True
	D False	E False	

106	A False	B False	C False
	D True	E False	

107	A False	B False	C True
	D False	E False	

108	A True	B False	C False
	D False	E True	

109	A False	B True	C False
	D False	E False	

110	A False	B False	C False
	D True	E False	

111	A True	B True	C False
	D True	E False	

112	A False	B False	C True
	D False	E True	

113	A False	B True	C False
	D True	E False	